Pregnancy After Preeclampsia

By Madison Lee

ISBN: 9781521115619

Two Pink Lines

I sit in the tiny bathroom of our ranch home, staring at the linoleum floor and listening to the rhythmic drip of the shower head. The face of the test turns dark as urine streams across it. I've never been a patient person, so turning away for the recommended three minutes, is absolute torture. I stare at the control line as it fills—dark pink. Suddenly, another line appears to its right. It is faint, but it's there.

Panic strikes. My heart begins to beat so intensely that I grab my chest, fearing a heart attack. My legs shake and I struggle to find my underwear. Once located, I quickly yank it up my legs before I pass out on the floor naked.

Shawn waits in the bedroom, just outside the door. I'm terrified to tell him, but unsure as to why. He is already an amazing father to his son, and will make a fantastic husband one day, but the fear weighs heavy on my soul. I grab the golden knob with my sweaty palm, but it's so drenched that I have to wipe it on my shirt before I'm able to open the door.

The television screen is the only light in the darkened bedroom. Shawn is waiting to greet me, and without a word, I hold the test in front of him. Immediately he lights up, and his face glows like a child's on Christmas morning. However, as much as I force it to, mine does not match. Actually, I'm struggling to hold back vomit. My hands tremble as I suck a deep breath through my nose to try and calm my nerves while blowing it out through pursed lips. I can't do

[1]

this; be a mom. His strong arms wrap around me as he hugs me to his chest. I melt into his embrace while endless thoughts course through my mind.

Six months. Six months is all we've been together and we're already pregnant. What if it doesn't work out? What if he leaves? I can't raise a baby alone. I don't even know how to change a diaper!

I lie on the bed. The breeze from the fan is starting to wick the moisture off my legs and it's causing me to shiver. I cover myself with a nearby blanket and hope the trembling will soon cease. Sleep will be a far-fetched goal now that it is five minutes until midnight. So, I stare at the television and zone out. Shawn lies beside me, running his fingers through my hair.

"It'll all be ok, babe," he whispers.

I want kids; I know I do. But, this is all happening faster than I expected. Apparently, I am extremely fertile, and apparently Shawn has good swimmers. I got pregnant without even trying, really. I thought it would take four to six months, at least. I was convinced I had time; time to prepare; time to research; time to decide if this is what I want. But, I guess my time is up.

I know neither of our parents will be on board with the whole thing. They had each made snide comments about it to us on previous occasions. Instructing Shawn to "keep it in his pants", and informing me that, "Shawn has no money to support more kids; he can barely pay for the one he has."

Well, obviously Shawn did not keep it in his pants, and I better be prepared to live frugally. Staring at the screen, my head goes crazy and thoughts pile up to a point of overflowing. My legs begin to tremble again as fear takes over and puddles of sweat form in every pore. Shawn texts on his phone next to me with a huge smile frozen on his face, unaware of the fact that I'm barely holding on to my sanity.

How bad could it be if it's making the man I love so happy?

I know my life is going to change drastically, but maybe it's not something to fear.

"Deep breaths, Ryan," I whisper to myself. "Deep breaths."

After a few hours of sleep, the sun illuminates the sky and I wait around until the offices open at the gynecologist. Dialing the number, I wonder if this is the correct move to make. Unfortunately, I don't have a **"Step-by-step guide to what to do when you find out you're pregnant"**, although it would be nice. Per usual, my hands are tiny slip-and-slides and my chest is tightening as the call connects and the phone rings. Once the secretary answers, I spout out nonsense that I'm hoping she understands.

"Pregnant. I am. Do you guys do that?"

What the hell am I saying? Hopefully she understands the words of my people.

"I'm sorry. Are you saying you're pregnant? If so, we can see you. Are you a new patient?"

"Yes. Wait, I mean no. I mean. I wasn't pregnant before now. So, I'm new for that, but I've been there before – you know, for my yearly visits."

Yearly visits means every so often when I have a UTI or pain in my ovary. I rarely went for a yearly. I probably haven't even seen the gynecologist in several years.

"Ok, well, you would be a new patient for our OBGYN doctors. When was your last period?"

"July 29th," I respond with certainty.

"Ok, so you are about six weeks along? We don't bring you in until ten weeks. Let me check the book for openings."

I respond brashly, "Ten weeks? Are you kidding me? I have to wait another month until I can validate that I have a tiny human growing inside me?"

The nurse does not appreciate my tone, but she chooses to ignore it instead of feeding into the charade.

"We have October 10th available?" she responds sternly, scolding me with her voice.

"Ok. I'm sorry for yelling at you," I respond. "Must be the hormones." My apology is half-hearted. "I will be there on the 10th."

"It's probably the hormones," she agrees. The phone clicks and the call is disconnected.

[3]

Well, Hello There Peanut

We sit in the waiting room for quite a while at the OBGYN's office. Doctors never seem to be on time, but I better get used to it. Over the course of my wait, several women walk through the doors with varying stomach sizes. They waddle from the desk and head straight into the bathroom to pee before even taking a seat. Every. Single. Time. Apparently, pregnancies cause mayhem on your bladder— just add it to the mental list of all the things I have to look forward to.

My hands begin to sweat again, so I wipe them on my jeans. Paranoid about what I've gotten myself into, my body begs me to flee. I feel the pounding of my heart as its pace increases, and my brain starts to turn foggy. Just as a panic attack begins to form, the nurse calls my name. It breaks me from my zone, and we follow her back to the exam room.

As I take a seat on the bed, and Shawn makes himself comfortable in a chair, a familiar face enters. She looks up from her paperwork after saying my name, and her smile fades. Realizing we went to high school together many moons ago, the awkwardness of the moment sets in.

Seeing acquaintances from my past is always weird. There's a reason I've excelled at staying out of contact all these years – I'm a professional at dodging social interactions. If I see someone in the grocery store, I hide in the light bulb aisle (because no one ever goes in that aisle anyway). Usually, they continue their shopping and never notice me. I don't have to engage in uncomfortable small talk, and I can just go about my life once the coast is clear. However, in this situation there is no light bulb aisle, and this is about to get downright uncomfortable.

"Take your bottoms off and lie down," she instructs in a cold tone.

I wink. "Are you hitting on me?"

She doesn't think it's funny.

Her face remains stoic. Embarrassment takes over and I do as she says, kicking myself for the previous sarcastic comment. Bedside manner must not have been her strong suit in nursing school.

A few moments later, the doctor busts through the door. His demeanor shifts the energy in the room from uncomfortable to just plain strange. A pair of blue overalls peak out under his white coat. In any other part of the country, it might be weird. But, we live in Pennsylvania, so...no, it's still weird.

After introducing himself, I immediately forget his name. I'm too nervous about the entire situation that I honestly couldn't care less about what to call him. I'm sure he will answer to "Doctor", anyway.

First, his cold and clammy hands start palpating my stomach. Upon finishing, he takes a seat on his chair and rolls down to the bottom of the bed. Staring in my eyes, he squirts lube onto the wand and inserts it into my vagina.

"It might be cold," he smirks.

I'm instantly uncomfortable. But, it's not the wand in my privates that's making me feel this way. There's something about the look on his face, or the way he makes eye contact with me for just a few seconds too long, that feels off. I chalk it up to me being young and naive. I'm sure this is all normal, besides, I don't have anything to compare it to considering I've never been pregnant before. All I know is that if I was in a bar, and a man stared at me that way, I would throw a drink in his face.

[6]

Men are lucky they don't have to deal with these things. In my opinion, it's insane that we allow complete strangers to do this to us. In fact, we pay them to. I am disgusted by it. Shawn had to wait at least a month for me to show him my lady bits, this guy got to see every minute detail within seconds.

Pulling myself out of my messy web of thoughts, I turn to the screen. Shawn stands at my head, his hand resting on my shoulder. As the seconds pass, silence deafens the room.

"Is everyth--- ?" I start.

"Ahh, there it is," he interrupts

"Really?" I question as the tears well up in my eyes.

The doctor nods his head and points to the tiny gray peanut on the screen. Up until this moment, I couldn't convince myself it was real. I had it in my head that there would be no baby. That the four tests I took were false positives and it was a fluke. In this moment, more emotions hit me than I expected.

"Do a lot of people cry?" I ask with an unsteady voice.

"Actually, no," Blair, my high school acquaintance, replies.

Man, what crawled up her ass? Did I offend her that badly with my wink? Lighten up.

I struggle to shut off the water works.

"Well, let's just blame it on pregnancy hormones, then." This has become my motto, and I am going to overuse the hell out of it.

After Dr. Overalls puts the wand away, I lower my legs and begin to sit up. Blair throws some paperwork at me on the first trimester of pregnancy.

"You'll have to come back in a month. I won't be seeing you again, though. You can schedule it at our other office closer to your home."

I'm not sure how to respond, so I simply nod my head and exit. "Thanks," I add, with zero emotion or eye contact.

Upon leaving the office, I stare at the ultrasound picture sitting on my lap. I don't feel that different. My stomach is still flat, and no one can tell I'm pregnant by looking at me.

[7]

Once home, I pass out within seconds of my butt hitting the couch, but I'm not really nauseous like everyone says I should be. For being ten weeks along already, this pregnancy has been a walk in the park.

I don't understand why women always complain so much; this is easy.

That evening, Shawn and I sit in the parking lot of the local pizza place, waiting to pick up our order. Next to us, a noticeably pregnant woman exits her car and walks by. Her waddle spurs envy that I didn't know I had. I want to hijack her belly; I want people to know that I am growing a human in my uterus. I want balloons and confetti thrown at me at all moments for how amazing I am because of this. I feel like I have done magic by creating a tiny human and now incubating it. It's an incredible gift, and I want every single person to know it.

But, there is no baby bump yet, and I have no idea when it will come. So, unless I want to pin a button to my shirt stating **I AM WITH CHILD,** I will have to live in the anonymity a little while longer. My maternity clothes that I picked up from the consignment shop are going to sit in my closet collecting dust, and now that I have concrete confirmation of the embryo, I'm not happy about it.

No One Likes Taking Tests

"It's a simple blood test," Doctor four in the practice explains while Shawn and I read over the pamphlet entitled **Quad screening test.**

My biggest pet peeve so far about my OBGYN decision is that I have to see a group of doctors. Every appointment is with a stranger. It bothers me so intensely, that I have considered switching practices, but at 15 weeks along, I feel like it's too late.

Today's doctor is an older man with gray hair. He was probably delivering Neanderthal babies in the Stone Age. I have to yell when I respond because his hearing is less than ideal. He sits on the stool and begins to explain about genetic testing; how it's an important tool they use to determine risk factors for a host of abnormalities.

"Trisomy 18, Trisomy 21, Spina Bifida, etc." he explained. "Because Shawn has Down syndrome on his side, I recommend the testing. It's something that you should be prepared for. In your case, it's a very real possibility."

I'm worried. I never thought about it before. One of Shawn's cousin's was born with Down syndrome and it does have a genetic link. This puts our future babies at an increased risk.

After briefly discussing this with the doctor, and amongst ourselves, we agree to the test.

"We can't do the test until 16 weeks. I'll write you a script. You can get the blood drawn at your local office and I'll have the results faxed here."

A week passes, and I'm sitting in the chair at our local clinic. A sweet nurse, wearing scrubs with dogs on them, draws several vials of blood from my arm.

"Your doctor should call you in about a week with the results. Keep the bandage on your arm for about 15 minutes to make sure the bleeding stops. Any questions?" she asks.

"No," I respond while pulling my sleeve down. I can feel the anxiety build as I think about raising a child with a disability. I ignorantly assumed my future children wouldn't be susceptible to abnormalities of any kind, but reality is setting in, and it's scary.

✳✳✳✳✳

Pregnancy is all about patience, of which I have none. This week of waiting is pure torture. Eight days have passed since my appointment when the phone finally rings. I answer it quickly.

"Hello!?" I blurt out.

"Hi, is this Ryan?"

"Yes," my voice shakes.

"Hi Ryan, this is Paula, a nurse from the OBGYN office. I'm calling to let you know that we have your blood results."

Yeah, I know why you're calling. Let's get to it.

"Yes? Is everything ok?" I rush her.

"The doctor would prefer that you come in," she informs.

"No," I respond. "I need you to tell me now, please."

I can hear the obvious hesitation in her voice.

"Well, as long as you understand that this is only one part of the test, and there's still more testing that needs to be done?" she asks.

"Yes, yes, I understand," I hurry her.

What is this chick waiting for? They are my results, so tell me.

"Well, unfortunately your bloodwork shows that the baby has a high probability of Down syndrome. We want you to come in to speak to a genetic counselor. We will do an ultrasound to check for certain markers. Once we validate the mutation, the counselor will be able to give you some information on Trisomy 21, and how you and your spouse can prepare yourselves for raising a child with disabilities."

I feel faint. Luckily I'm already sitting down, or I might pass out. My heart pounds in my chest and sweat floods from every pore of my body. My eyes cloud over as the walls begin closing in. Noises in the background become distant and I struggle to swallow. I'm aware of what's forming.

A panic attack. I am having a panic attack. I think to myself, trying to mentally prepare.

Deep breaths, Ryan. Get a hold of yourself. The baby needs oxygen. You can't pass out.

I pull the hair band on my wrist and let it go. The metal clasp snaps hard. The pain rips me out of the attack and forces me back to reality.

Shawn stares at me from across the table waiting for words to jump from my mouth to his ears. Upon locking eyes, he knows something is wrong. The chair falls over from the sheer speed that he forces it back. Rushing to my side, he holds me in his arms.

"What is it? What's wrong?"

I hand him the phone.

"Hello? Yes, this is Shawn. Can you tell me what you told my fiancée?"

He listens for a few moments. As she fills him in, his mouth drops and his face turns a ghostly white.

"Ok, we will see you Tuesday. Thank you."

[11]

He shakes his head and hangs up the phone. Taking a moment to gather his emotions, he picks me up and carries me to the couch. For a few minutes, we are both silent.

"It just makes our baby even more special," he tells me as he wipes the tears from my cheeks. "It will be ok."

✳✳✳✳✳

The next day, I spend hours researching. I read testimonials from parents of children with Down syndrome, along with any article I can get my hands on. Every piece of information helps me rationalize it. I like to be prepared–it eases my anxiety. As the knowledge fills my head, I begin to accept our future. Most children with D.S. live very fulfilling lives. Some are able to work and drive, and a select few live on their own. I will remain optimistic and open-minded going into this.

Before our appointment, I prepare a list of questions for the doctor and the genetic counselor.

"Ryan? You and Shawn can come back now."

At almost twenty weeks, they decide to do the anatomy scan to check the baby's growth, and the second portion of the quad screen in one visit. I roll down the elastic on my maternity pants and let out a wide tooth grin as my baby bump is unveiled. At last! I am visibly pregnant and extremely proud.

"Ok, the gel will be cold. I'm sorry. Let's get started," the tech explains with a sympathetic smile.

She is young—twenty-two, maybe. I say young—even though she's realistically around my age. The energy in the room is strange, as if she knows about our special baby. I don't want sympathy. I don't look at it as something that deserves that. My baby is not a charity case, and I don't think it should be treated as one.

After a moment of silence, she begins the scan. First, she measures the baby's head.

"It's very large," she explains, "measuring about 3-4 weeks ahead of where it should be."

"What does that mean?" Shawn asks. "Is that bad? It sounds bad."

He reaches his hand out to hold my thigh, his eyes begging for answers.

"Not necessarily. The doctor will let you know more," she responds without shifting her gaze from the screen. Continuing on, she then measures its arms, abdomen, and legs.

"I'm going to check the fluid behind the neck now," she states.

Shawn and I know what that means from our hours of research. The nuchal-fold is considered a hard marker for D.S. if it contains more fluid than normal. We prepare ourselves for what we already know she will find and begin nodding our heads awaiting the information.

"It's within normal range," the tech explains, surprised. "There are other things I need to check, though."

She looks puzzled, but continues on with the scan.

"I'm going to examine the placenta and blood flow. I'm printing out some pictures for you guys as I go along."

My head is busting at the seams with questions I desperately need answers to.

Why is the baby's head so big but the fluid normal? Does it have Down syndrome? Why doesn't this tech know anything? Why is she pushing so hard on my bladder?

"Do you want to know the gender?" she interrupts my endless thoughts.

Shawn and I know it's a girl, without a doubt. We had a name picked out a week after the stick turned pink. There was never a question in our minds; it was just something we subconsciously believed.

"Sure," I respond.

"It's a girl," she says, in the most cheerful voice she can muster.

[13]

"Duh," I blurt out. "I'm sorry, I didn't mean that. We just had a gut feeling. We already have a name and everything."

She awkwardly smiles and hands me the print outs. "I'm going to have the doctor look at the scans. He will probably be in to go over a few things."

She leaves the room and I immediately turn to Shawn, my lips unable to hold back the words that have been dying to get out. "The nuchal-fold is normal? What does that mean? But, her head is huge?"

Shawn shakes his head, "I'm not sure what it all means, babe. Let's see what the doctor says."

I've never been a patient person. It's definitely one of my downfalls and it annoys me how impatient I can be. Shawn is the opposite—he could wait years for an answer of something and remain content. It's one trait about him that drives me crazy and yet I find myself envying it right now.

Tapping fingers on my belly, I wait for the doctor. Wait, wait, wait.

After twenty minutes, he knocks on the door. I quickly change my disgust to a cheerful smile as he enters. Let's face it—he has the answers I desperately crave, so I can't greet him with a snarl.

"Let's take a look here. Do you mind?"

He motions to my belly. I nod my head and slide my pants back down. Millions of questions begin to multiply in my head as worry once again seizes all thoughts.

Why would he need to look? Something major is wrong. He's afraid to tell us.

I squeeze Shawn's hand so hard that I can feel him flinch.

He repeats the scans that the tech already preformed. He measures her head, nuchal-fold, arms, legs, and stomach.

Why not just tell us she has Down syndrome and send us to the genetic counselor? What's with the secrecy and the duplicate scans? I don't understand. What is wrong with our baby?

[14]

Infinite hours of waiting occur as he silently stares at the screen, scrutinizing the gray and white areas and conducting more measurements without saying a word.

Finally, he speaks, "Did the tech tell you the gender?"

"A girl," Shawn and I respond in unison.

He wipes the gel from my stomach and returns the wand to the desk.

"Ok," he starts with a deep breath. "Well, your baby seems healthy. Her head is measuring ahead by a pretty significant amount, but she has no other markers for Trisomy 21."

A surprised sigh exits my lips.

"However," he interrupts. "There is something wrong with the placenta. I'll have the counselor explain more."

"What do you mean, 'there's something wrong'?" I ask with obvious nerves that cause my voice to tremble. "Is everything going to be ok?"

"It's hard to say," he responds. "I need to read over your genetic testing. Why don't you meet with the counselor while I do that?"

I'm pissed.

How do you not know? What kind of doctor are you?

I keep my mouth shut as Shawn drags me out of the room and into the counselor's office. Her chipper attitude is misplaced.

Why are you so happy knowing people are seeing you after receiving news about issues with their baby? You're in the wrong profession, have some damn compassion.

I want to put her head through a wall, but I know that's just the hormones talking—I think.

"Please, take a seat. Now, according to your genetic screening, you tested high on the probability of the baby having Trisomy 21, or Down syndrome. However, after your scan, the doctor has concluded that we were mistaken in reading the screening. Instead, you have an issue with your placenta. Apparently, we are learning that placental issues show the same as Down syndrome on the blood test. Instead, you are at high risk for Preeclampsia."

Shawn and I have mentally prepared ourselves to raise a child with D.S. We had accepted it and were excited about the journey. Now, we are back at square one. Tears flow down my cheeks, and I feel like I've lost something. It's hard to explain exactly, but it is disheartening learning that the baby is ok after being convinced she wasn't.

Shawn wraps his arm around my shoulders and pulls me into him. "It's good news, babe."

"Is it?" I wonder. "What kind of things do we need to worry about with this Preeclampsia? Is it dangerous?"

"I'm going to give you a pamphlet on the signs and symptoms to watch for. We are going to schedule a 24 hour urine test to get your base levels of protein. The doctor wants you to start on a daily dose of blood thinner to maintain good blood flow through the placenta. If you have an unrelenting headache, severe edema, vision changes, pain in the upper right quadrant, or high blood pressure, call the doctor immediately. Preeclampsia is very dangerous to you and the baby."

I begin to panic. "Am I going to lose the baby?" I cry. "Is this life-threatening?"

The lady's smile fades as she shakes her head. "Plenty of women go on to have a healthy baby even with Preeclampsia. You just need to monitor the symptoms and stay on top of things. Everything should be fine. Now that the doctors are aware of your condition, we will monitor you and your baby more closely. You will attend regular scans and NST's, or non-stress tests, throughout the remainder of your pregnancy. We will set you up with a Perinatologist for those."

We leave the office with more questions than answers. I still believe I am carrying a baby with D.S. and that the doctors are idiots. Scans are unreliable, and blood tests can be misread. Erring on the side of caution, I follow their advice and stop for blood thinners on the way home.

After sharing the news with our families, we proceed to researching. For the next few weeks, we educate ourselves on every bit of information we can find, which isn't very much. Unfortunately, there is very little known about the complication, and very little research on it. I join groups on social media of moms who have been through it; I read articles published on blogs and studies performed by medical students, but I'm left terrified and unprepared. The only truth I'm sure of, is that it can result in maternal and fetal death, and really shouldn't be taken lightly.

"Did you know that it can be deadly? I can die, baby can die..." I yell while I stand in the middle of the living room.

Shawn looks up from his phone.

"The only cure is delivery. They have no idea why it happens or what causes it. And, there's no way to prevent it in future pregnancies or to stop it from happening or progressing," I continue.

He coaxes me over to the couch, pulling me into his arms. "I'm scared, too, babe," he whispers.

Future pregnancies.

I always knew I wanted two kids by the time I was thirty. Now, I need to focus on making it out of this pregnancy alive— getting both of us out alive. So many things change in an instant without notice and constant panic attacks are making it impossible to sleep.

Maintenance Leads to Emergency

If you've never done a 24-hour urine collection test, you're lucky. They've made me do it multiple times, and every time proves more annoying than the last. In brief, you have to collect every drop of urine you excrete within a 24-hour period. You pee in a cup that hooks onto your toilet seat, dump it in a carton and store it in your refrigerator. Yup, your big jug-o-pee sits right next to your chocolate milk.

Then, you nonchalantly carry your urine jug to the doctor and set it down next to you on the floor of the waiting room. If you're lucky, people won't realize what's inside of it, but I'm not that lucky.

Once you hand it over, they send it to the lab for testing. If your protein levels are over 300, you're in the danger zone.

I am now closing in on about 34 weeks pregnant and waddle into the waiting room holding my full jug of urine. The Perinatologist had requested weekly 24-hour urine scans, and I dream about the day that I will finish peeing and simply flush it down.

After dropping off my urine with the nurse, I head to the exam room for my ultrasound.

"Hi Ryan," the tech says cheerfully. They have all become extremely friendly after seeing me so often.

"Hey," I respond with a smile.

The tech prepares the wand with gel and coasts it over my giant belly. I watch as our little girl's profile appears on the screen. Shawn's face gleams upon seeing her, and I am quick to match.

"Ok, the baby looks good. Her head is still measuring about 3-4 weeks ahead, but otherwise healthy. Let's check the placenta, quick."

I watch her scan the placenta. She listens to the blood flow and adds color to the screen to demonstrate the circulation through it and the umbilical cord. After a few moments, her smile fades.

"Ok. I'm going to go tell the doctor. He will want to look at it and decide where to go from here," she tells us with an unsure voice.

I can feel the panic build. They had always said I may have issues with the placenta, but it seems that now my fears are becoming a reality.

Something is failing. Something is wrong. Why don't these people tell me anything? Why do they always leave the room when something is wrong? I hate secrets.

I sit up and cannot stop my legs from trembling. A wave of nausea hits me, and I suck a deep breath through my nose to try and force it back down.

"Deep breaths, babe. Don't panic until we know what's going on," Shawn comforts me as we wait.

An agonizing ten minutes pass before the doctor decides to enter. I have successfully talked myself down from a panic attack, only to feel the rise of it again upon seeing the Doctor. His face is troubled, and he rushes over to the machine, hurrying me to lie back.

"Sorry," he mumbles. "It's been very busy today. A lot of emergencies."

You're not making me feel any better here, Doc.

He scans my belly, heading straight to the placenta. After a few moments of studying, he clears his throat.

"There's some pretty major issues with blood flow," he begins. "It's what we were worried about but it doesn't mean we have to deliver yet. I'm going to move the scans to twice a week, and I'll have your regular OB check your urine and blood pressure once a week. We will keep that baby in as long as we can, but I doubt very much that you will make it to full-term."

Nerves soar through my body and tunnel vision takes over as I sit up. I'm struggling to get a deep breath as my lungs refuse to function.

"Should I be afraid? Because I am afraid," I cry. "Are we going to be ok?"

The doctor looks me square in the eye while holding both of my hands. "I'm going to take care of you and your baby, Ryan. We will take it one day at a time."

There's the Pre-e

"156 over 92," the nurse reads aloud.

"Take it again," the female doctor demands. She is the only one in the practice that I have liked so far. I have two left to meet over the last five weeks of my pregnancy, but I'm hoping she's the one to deliver our baby.

"153 over 91," the nurse proclaims.

"That's not good," the doctor mumbles. "Have you been having any other symptoms? Blurry vision, headaches, swelling?"

"Well, I'm pretty swollen," I say as I point to my feet, lifting my jeans. "I can't fit in sneakers anymore. Thank goodness it's been a mild spring; otherwise I would be in trouble."

She pushes on my feet with her finger and the indent temporarily holds. "Pitting edema," she shakes her head.

"You're Preeclamptic. But, there is no significant protein in your urine yet. I want you to lie back for about ten minutes and we will recheck your blood pressure. When is your next appointment with the Perinatologist?" she asks.

"Wednesday," I respond.

"Ok. Well, if you feel progressively worse between now and then, you need to call me. I'm worried about you, and this can progress pretty rapidly. You need to stay aware of your symptoms."

Fear doesn't even begin to describe what I'm feeling as I'm lying on the table awaiting the nurse's return. The paper crinkles under me as I struggle to find comfort and halt my shaking muscles.

My blood pressure will never lower if I can't calm myself down.

I close my eyes and try to find a positive thought to comfort me through visualization.

Hot sand under your toes, Ryan. Crashing waves against the shore. Breathe in the salty air and listen to the seagulls scream as they coast through the sky.

"137 over 88," the nurse shares aloud.

The doctor peeks in from the hall. "Ok, she can go home. Make sure she has all the info on symptoms and our number for the emergency line."

I don't want to leave. I don't feel safe leaving. Something in me wants to stay; begs me to stay. I feel like going home is a horrible decision that every cell in my body is fighting, but I take the paper the nurse hands me and head out the door.

Once home, I decide to pack my hospital bag. Staring at my swollen feet, I question if I'll make it through the night.

"One," I count a kick as I sit on the bed to rest. Another rumble scoots across my stomach, "two".

Within eight minutes, I feel ten kicks and am relieved that, even though my body is failing, she's doing just fine.

Propping my feet up on a diaper box, I read through the pamphlet they gave me on Preeclampsia symptoms.

Most babies will survive if born beyond 32 weeks gestation.

A sigh sneaks through my lips. A small sense of relief sets in knowing that even if we have to deliver her, and she will be premature, there's a good chance she will survive.

Preeclampsia can cause fetal and maternal mortality.

[24]

I read over the words again, this time aloud, "fetal and maternal mortality."

My legs tremble so hard that they fall off the box.

Shawn peeks in from the hallway and notices my panic attack growing.

"I -- I can't breathe."

He rushes to my side and picks up the pamphlet that has fallen from my hand.

"Mortality. Mortality!" I yell through short huffs of air.

Shawn shoves the pamphlet in his mouth and picks me up off the bed. Carrying me to the couch, he lies me down and kisses me on the forehead.

"Let's talk about this," he starts.

"It says we can die, babe. Me, her, both of us!"

Tears form in his eyes as he pushes his hat off his forehead and plays with the tiny strands of blonde hair that fall out. The hand he's rubbing my shin with becomes slightly sticky, and it's the first time I've seen this much worry in his face. I'm almost relieved to know he's panicking, too.

"I won't let that happen!" he yells. "That can't happen."

The sounds of our muffled cries encompass the room as we allow every emotion to exit our bodies. The fear is real, and it's suffocating us. We need to find a way to get through this and to make it out alive.

Day One

My swollen and crusty eyes open to the morning sun, and I'm thankful we made it through the night. I flip the pen open and cross yesterday off the calendar.

"Tuesday, April 7th. Today I'm 36 weeks," I say to myself as a content smile holds steady on my face. Only four weeks left to go.

Because of yesterday's symptoms, I take it easy for a good portion of the day—cleaning up here and there and doing a few loads of laundry. Shawn is working until seven, so by 3:00 pm when I decide to rest, I know it's only a few more hours that I have to be alone.

I hate being alone.

Around five, I decide to take a shower, hoping the warm water will calm my aching feet. While washing my hair, an intense headache begins. It comes on hard and feels as if someone is pulling each piece of hair from my head, strand by strand. The only thing I can compare it to, is the worst case of hat hair I've ever had, multiplied by a million.

Is this the headache the doctor was talking about?

No, it has to be a coincidence. My vision is fine, and I have no chest pain. I exit the shower and dry off, hurrying to read the pamphlet of symptoms again.

A headache that does not fade with pain medication.

I pop two pain pills to see if it helps. Unable to keep calm, I pace the floor and watch the minutes tick by, one by one.

After a grueling hour passes, the pain intensifies. Tears are now forming in my eyes as I dial Mom's number.

"Ryan?" she asks with worry. "Is everything alright?"

I'm unable to speak, and instead, blubbers of tears fill the silence.

"I'm on my way."

I text Shawn at work and wait for a call back; he can't have his cell phone on while he's on the line, so it might be a while. Staring out the window, I deal with the constant symptoms of a panic attack before Mom finally pulls in the driveway. Barely putting the car in park, she sprints to the door.

"What's wrong?" she asks, concerned.

"I—I I'm scared," I cry. "My head. And, my feet are—"

She grabs the phone from my hand and walks inside, instructing me to sit on the couch as she dials the number.

"Let's call the doctor. I think you need to go to the hospital," Mom insists.

The answering service receives the call and Mom briefs them on my situation. Within a few minutes, we receive a call back. My favorite doctor is on the other end.

"Tell me what's going on," she mutters. "Did your symptoms get worse? Anything new?"

I feel like I'm bothering her. She probably has emergencies she should be taking care of, so I try to make it quick.

"I was in to see you yesterday with signs of Preeclampsia— I don't know if you remember me. Well, for the last couple of hours, I have been having an intense headache that isn't fading with the pain meds."

She doesn't hesitate to respond. "Go to the ER right away. I will meet you there. I will let them know you are coming. I want you admitted right away."

I click to end the call. Fear engulfs me as I slump to the floor. Every ounce of my body shuts down as the world turns black. Mom wraps her arms around me, coaching me through the attack as my phone rings. It's Shawn. She pulls it from my hand and fills him in, juggling my emotions simultaneously.

I can hear the worry in his voice from across the room.

"I'll meet you there. Tell her I love her," he yells through the speaker.

✸✸✸✸✸

I zone out in the passenger seat as the yellow line on the highway turns blurry. My contacts are so muddled from the tears, that it's impossible to tell if my vision has been affected. I snap the hair band on my arm until my wrist is sore. I can't keep the panic at bay any longer.

"It'll be ok," Mom assures me as she places her palm on my thigh.

Dad reaches forward from the back seat, resting his hand on my shoulder. "We are here, sweetheart. It's all going to be ok, now."

"I'm scared," I mumble through chattering lips. "What if something happens?"

Tightness fills my chest, and an all-too-familiar feeling begins to rule my body. A panic attack is forming, and I don't have the strength to stop it. My hearing muffles and tunnel vision fills my eyes. Mom squeezes my leg with one hand as she uses the other to hold the wheel.

"Everything will be ok, Ryan. I'm here. Deep breaths, remember?"

Of course I remember. It's just not working anymore.

Sitting at the entrance, my headache is unbearable. Tiny needles stab my skull and my eyes hurt from the tears. I feel like I'm dreaming and death's knocking on the door. My parents' voices are distant and incoherent even though they are only inches away. Dad runs to get a nurse while Mom helps me out of the car.

There are only a few people in the ER, and a nurse greets me with a wheelchair at the door. I thankfully take a seat, relieving pressure from my inflated feet.

"Are you Ryan?" another nurse calls from the doors.

"Yes, she is!" Mom yells from behind, tossing the keys to Dad and instructing him to park the car.

"Come on back. Your doctor called us."

I rub my head attempting to ease the pain. For a moment, I question if it's the "right" kind of headache that they've been explaining. I'm still not experiencing the upper quadrant pain, and my urine was fine at the appointment yesterday. Maybe I'm wrong and overreacting — perhaps it's not Preeclampsia.

Mom fills out paperwork while the nurse wheels me to the intake room. She follows behind, digging an insurance card from my purse.

"I'm going to take your blood pressure to see where we are at."

I relax my arm and she tightens the cuff. As it fills, my head throbs and my heart beats in my fingers, toes, lips, and eyes.

This can't be a good sign.

"Oh," she says. "Let me page your OBGYN and see what she wants to do. These numbers are very high."

Mom leans over to look at the machine.

"I would assume they would want to keep her!" she exclaims. "Why is this even a question with numbers that high?"

I stare at her. I don't need to hear the results— I know I'm in a danger zone. Mom tails the nurse out of the room, making sure she follows through on admitting me.

I wait, alone. Dad is parking the car. Mom is glued to the nurse's hip, and I'm still waiting for Shawn to arrive. I can feel Blake kicking in my belly. That's what we decided to name her: Blake. I can't believe that she is going to be in my arms this soon—a month early.

I focus on a moment to enjoy the feeling of her tiny body moving inside of me, just in case it's the last day that I'll be able

[30]

to. With a deep breath, I let out a tired moan and lay my hands on my stomach in the shape of a heart.

"Stay strong in there little one. Mommy loves you," I whisper.

"Ok, we are going to admit you. They want to do an induction. Your blood pressure is too high to risk. You'll do a urine test in triage to see where your protein is. The only treatment now, is to get your baby out; sooner rather than later," the nurse explains while Mom brushes the hair out of my eyes.

My body shakes in fear. I'm sweating and shivering in unison. As I adjust myself in the wheelchair attempting to find comfort, warm hands push down on my shoulders.

"Hey, babe," Shawn says as he kisses my cheek. "How are you feeling?"

Perfect timing.

I can feel the tension release from my body immediately. Nothing can go wrong now that he's here.

I fail to answer without crying. He stares into my worried eyes and wraps his invincible arms around me. The panic attack is immediately subsiding for the first time in hours.

"Just think, soon you'll get to meet our baby. Try to focus on that, and not worry about the in-between. It will all work out."

Shawn and I were always a good pair. He's very grounded and laid back. He doesn't panic or get emotional— he just looks at things for exactly what they are. He keeps me from reaching insanity every single day. And, I couldn't possibly thank God enough.

They wheel me to labor and delivery, and we sit in the hallway outside of triage for over an hour. My head throbs. Shawn and Mom peek in the nursery at the newborns with their tiny hats and blankets, but I can't muster the energy to join them.

"Ryan? You can come on back. We are ready for you."

Once in triage, I immediately change into a gown and pee in a cup. After taking a seat on the bed, a blonde nurse hooks me up to an IV and a fetal monitor. A few moments later, a tiny Asian woman enters.

[31]

"Hello Ryan, I am Doctor Miller. I'm going to start an induction on you. First, we are going to try and ripen your cervix so it begins to dilate."

I nod my head, even though I have no clue what this entails.

She walks over to my IV bags and reads the labels. "Ok, we need to start you on the magnesium right away to try and get your blood pressure under control for delivery."

I had read about the magnesium in one of the pamphlets the Perinatologist gave me. There are a lot of side effects that come along with it, but it's essential for keeping blood pressure under control during Preeclampsia. I know it isn't an option; it's a necessity.

As Dr. Miller describes the drugs that will soften and then dilate my cervix, the nurse hangs the magnesium.

Almost instantly, I realize that it is liquid hell.

My face is the first thing to feel the wrath when my cheeks inflame like severe sunburn. I feel nauseous, drowsy, and flu-like. It's enough to make me want to rip the needle out of my skin, and give up on all of it, but I push forward. I know I need the magnesium to stay alive and to keep my baby alive, but it's close to unbearable.

About an hour into it, an intense stomach ache hits me out of nowhere. I need to use the bathroom, and quickly. I rush to sit up, and struggle to pull my backless gown over my bare butt. Modesty is important to me— I don't want to be exposed.

Due to the size of the tiny room, I can't bring my IV hanger in with me and am forced to leave it right outside the door. As I sit on the toilet, I can't control the humiliating bowel movement that is coming.

Shawn and my parents sit only a few feet away, quietly chatting through the open door. I can't hold back the inevitable, as much as I want to. The magnesium has destroyed my intestinal tract and it needs to come out. Closing my eyes in the hopes that I become invisible, I relax my muscles and let it go.

"Whoa, everything ok in there?" Shawn laughs.

I'm humiliated. The nurse peeks through the door.

"Are you ok, sweetie?" she asks. "Blame it on the magnesium; it's a laxative."

[32]

I push out a smile and stare at the open door. Mom walks over and tries to force it closed, but the cords and wires refuse to allow it.

After a while, my stomach is empty and I feel a little better. After returning to the bed, Shawn reaches for my hand.

"I'm sorry you aren't feeling well, babe. Is there anything I can do to help?"

I smack my lips. "My mouth is really dry. Could you get me something to drink?"

"No," the nurse blurts out. "Nothing to drink. She's getting her hydration through the IV. She could aspirate if she goes into surgery. Nothing by mouth."

The idea of not being able to drink anything worries me. My mouth immediately craves water with an intensity I've never had before upon hearing the news.

"Once your cervix is ripened, we will insert a Foley ball and inflate it. It will help you dilate. After we get that in, we will put you on Pitocin to intensify contractions and speed it along."

I agree to all of it; no questions asked.

✳✳✳✳✳

Throughout the night, my cervix ripens enough to start dilating. I try to sleep, but nerves and anxiousness are keeping me awake. Now that I'm on the magnesium, and my blood pressure has dropped a little, my headache has subsided. The majority of my time is spent sitting around, waiting for the blood pressure cuff to fill every half hour while staring blankly at the television.

Around 3:00am, the resident inserts a Foley bulb. It's uncomfortable and creates a sensation of fullness in my vagina along with some random, sharp pains. But, it is all part of the process, and I'm sure what I'm feeling is completely normal.

Shawn left to run Dad home, and Mom is resting on the chair in the corner. I scroll around on my phone while I wait for something—anything—to happen.

Boredom is exhausting and mind numbing. I had worked labor up in my mind for so long, that it's been disappointing thus far.

[33]

I thought I would start with the medication, have a few hours' worth of contractions, and push our daughter out by morning. I'm quickly realizing that this is not going to be how it is in the movies.

Sometime in the early morning hours, I don't meet my daughter— instead, I meet Pitocin. Within moments, I realize that magnesium was nothing compared to the liquid hell that comes along with this nasty drug.

Random light contractions turn hard and strong in a matter of minutes. I go from smiling and talking, to moaning out in pain. No position is comfortable, and I'm starting to lose my strength.

After about an hour of breathing through unrelenting pain, I beg the nurse for help. "Is there anything I can have for relief?"

"It's too early for an epidural, since you're only at about two centimeters. You can have Stadol. It just goes in your IV," she offers.

I nod my head, and she calls the order down to the pharmacy. A half-hour later, she's hanging the bag and I'm singing her praises.

I regret my decision instantly while I struggle to breathe.

My lungs and throat are closing; it must be an allergic reaction.

I call to the nurse who is standing with her back to me, talking on the phone.

"I can't breathe. I can't breathe," I repeat in a whisper.

She glances at me, rolls her eyes, and returns to her conversation.

Mom screams, "She says she can't breathe! Hang up the damn phone and get your ass over here!"

The nurse meanders over. "Her oxygen levels are fine. See? That's what this finger device measures. There's nothing wrong besides what's in her head."

She walks away, picking the phone off the counter without another word.

"She clicked it off," Mom informs. "She stopped the drugs. I think it's for the best. Apparently, she doesn't want to do her job anyway."

Mom fixes the pillow behind my head as Shawn rubs my feet.

"What time is your shift over?" Mom asks the nurse.

"An hour," she responds.

"Good," Mom says, coldly.

Day Two

It's Wednesday—late afternoon, I think. In the hospital, it's hard to keep track of the time. I have finally moved out of triage and into a delivery room. Contractions are intense, and without relief, my body is running on empty. I still haven't seen my OB, but the resident has returned to check my progress.

"She's at four. She can get an epidural if she needs to," she explains to Shawn. "It'll help her rest. She still has a long way to go."

I overhear and nod my head with enthusiasm. "Yes, please. I need to sleep."

"I'll let the anesthesiologist know and put you on the list. It could be a little while, we are pretty busy."

A sigh escapes. I never really had expectations about what I want during delivery. I know I don't want a mirror, and I know I want skin to skin when she is born, but that's all I'm adamant about. I'll be the first to admit that I am naive, clueless, and unprepared going into this— especially a month early. I have put every ounce of faith in my doctors and nurses and it's given me a false sense of security.

I'm in pain for two more excruciating hours before the epidural arrives. I am exhausted and delirious. I've been here awhile, but have no clue how long.

"Hold still," the anesthesiologist scolds me. "Do you want to be paralyzed?"

No. No, I don't want to be paralyzed.

"I'm sorry. I'm just having a contraction," I whine.

"I don't care. If you don't stay still, I could really do some damage. Your tattoo is making this very difficult."

I cry in my pillow as the contractions continue and I struggle to remain still, sitting on the edge of the bed. The nurse counts me through them as the young anesthesiologist struggles to shove the needle into my spine. Every time I flinch, he lets out a huff of anger onto the back of my neck.

I drop my forehead on to the nurse's shoulder. "You're doing great, Ryan. He's almost done," she whispers.

She is my favorite person in the whole world at the moment; a blonde angel sent to save me from labor. She pats my head with a cool cloth and rubs my shoulders with her soft hands. Her compassion is incomparable.

Once the needle is placed and the catheter for the epidural is in, relief is instant. It isn't exactly what I expected, though. I still have full function of both my legs, even though the pain is substantially less. I close my eyes, and within minutes I fall asleep for the first time in 24 hours.

Mom and Shawn follow suit, and we all get some much deserved slumber.

A few hours later, I'm awakened by painful contractions. I push the button on my epidural, praying that an extra dose of medicine will offer some relief. Unfortunately, it doesn't. My blonde angel, Amy, is standing by my side in the dim lit room. Shawn and Mom are still sleeping in the corner.

"Are you feeling them again?" she asks with her eyes fixated on the screen.

I wince in pain. "Yes and pretty severely."

[38]

"I'll call the anesthesiologist," she says. "You shouldn't be feeling them."

As she hangs up the line, the resident meanders through the door for another cervix check. A hoard of students follows her, holding notepads in their hands. They each grab a pair of gloves out of the box that hangs on the wall, eager to get in on the action.

I hesitantly open my legs for the entire room to see. A male student in his twenties stares at me from the back of the group. I try to push the blanket down to cover myself, and the resident senses my insecurity.

"You're still only about five," she explains while she covers my vagina with the blanket. "I'm going to break your water and see if we can get things moving. If not, we need to consider a C-section. I'll give you a few more hours."

I don't want a C-section.

Keeping my panic disorder under control during major surgery would be an incredible feat that I don't want to have to partake in. But, if push comes to shove, I will do it if I have to.

"Ok," is the only response I can muster.

"I'm going to put a call into your OB and just let them know where you're at. I also want to do some bloodwork again to check all your levels."

Shawn had awoken during my exam and is now by my side for the pain of the contractions. It has been days since I've had anything to eat, but the thing I want more than anything in the world? A damn drink.

"Dry mouth?" Amy asks while I smack my lips together.

"Yes, it's awful."

"It's another side effect of the magnesium. Chew on some ice chips, it'll help."

I place ice chips in my mouth— so many ice chips that I can no longer feel my tongue, but nothing is quenching my thirst. I crave water.

"Can I please have something to drink?" I beg.

[39]

Amy smiles but shakes her head. "Nothing to drink, just ice chips. You're getting your hydration through the IV."

I set them on the window ledge, praying that the sun will melt the ice so that I can drink the water. I daydream about giant pools filled with lemonade and swimming in a sea of iced tea as my mouth begs me for something—anything to calm the desire.

What a bitch. So much for being my favorite nurse. Maybe she can't understand what I am saying because my tongue has dried up in my mouth and turned to dust.

I turn to Shawn and begin to weep.

"Babe, I'm so thirsty," I cry.

His face changes from empathy to determination. He holds the cup in his masculine hands, trying to melt the ice with his body heat.

"Can she just have some water? A few sips?"

Amy shakes her head again. "No, I'm sorry."

Mom begins fiercely digging in her purse on the windowsill. "Try this, it might help," she instructs as she hands me a piece of gum.

Chewing obnoxiously loud just to annoy Amy, the gum does very little to combat my thirst. I consider crying and drinking my tears as they run down my cheeks, but I'm too angry to create any.

An hour later, the resident returns.

"I'm here to check you again. I'm going to check you every hour for a little while. If you don't start progressing soon, my advice is to do a C-section," the resident explains. "I personally would do it now, but your OB is fighting me on it."

The anesthesiologist walks in during the exam. It's a woman this time, and she has a very intimidating resting-bitch-face.

"What's going on here?" she blurts out. Amy brings her up to speed while I have the resident's fingers in my cervix.

"The epidural seems to have fallen out? It isn't working to combat her pain any longer. We wanted you to take a look."

[40]

As I haphazardly lay on the bed with my vagina exposed to the entire room, and everyone talks about me— rather than to me— millions of thoughts run through my mind.

Thank goodness I shaved in the shower yesterday. Wait, was that yesterday? How many days ago was that? How long have I been here? What time of day is it? It's dark outside, right? Is it nighttime? What is this doctor's name again? Will she be the one who delivers my baby? Why do I even have an OB if they are never here?

"She's still at 5," she explains to Amy. "Your OB is here now; he just finished an emergency cesarean. I'm going to have him come in," she continues talking as she removes her blue gloves and throws them in the garbage can by the door. "I think we are going to move forward with a C-section. Let me check your bloodwork, and I'll be right back."

I fix my gown and blankets. All of the modesty I once had has been stripped from my soul and tossed in the garbage cans that are filled with dirty gloves. The anesthesiologist huffs at me as she pushes on my back, urging me forward.

"Damn thing fell out," she grumbles. "I have to redo it."

How the heck does it just fall out? Was it something I did? How could it be? I've been lying in this bed for four years not moving and dreaming about drinking a swimming pool, it couldn't have been my fault.

"I'll need to put a new one in," she explains. "Is this what you want?"

"Yes, please," I respond without hesitation.

Of course I want the epidural. I am only at five centimeters. There's no way I could handle this without it.

Amy directs Shawn and Mom out of the room as they place my second epidural. While clutching my pillow, I lean in to her for support.

"Are you being abused in your home? Are you afraid of anyone you're living with?" Amy whispers in my ear.

What? Seriously? I'm in the middle of a contraction, with a complete stranger stabbing me in the spine. I have been in labor for who knows how many days, and you're wondering if I'm getting beat up at home? This is your protocol?

I sit back and stare directly into her soul.

"No."

"Ok," she responds. "I just wanted to make sure."

Shawn and Mom return with sandwiches, but are unsure about whether they should eat them in front of me. I really don't care; hunger is the last thing I'm feeling.

A nurse flings open the door. "Her potassium is bottoming out. She needs some ASAP. Send an order down," she yells, frantically.

Amy dials the phone. "I need potassium, stat."

Across the room, Shawn and Mom drop their sandwiches and rush to my side.

"What does that mean?"

"Try not to panic," Amy begins. "It means she could go into cardiac arrest if we don't bring her levels up. Sometimes it's a side effect of the magnesium. It's not something to mess with. This is serious."

Twenty minutes pass, and no potassium bag has arrived. Mom paces the floor while Shawn stands at my head, dabbing a cool rag on my neck trying to keep my panic disorder under control.

"Tell me where the damn shit is and I'll go get it myself!" Mom yells.

"In the basement. Suite B22. I'll call and let them know you're coming," Amy directs.

"This is absolutely fucking ridiculous!" she yells from the hall.

Ten minutes later, Mom returns with the bag.

"I don't want to do a C-section on her yet," my OB explains to the resident. "Give her some more time. I can't put her through the stress until her potassium is stable. In about an hour, I want you to up her Pitocin."

[42]

The resident storms out of the room. "You're going to kill them!" she yells.

Kill us? The statement bounces around in my head. I am scared, and I can tell by the look on Shawn's face, that he is too. I grip his hand.

"Are you having a contraction, babe?"

Surprisingly, I'm not sure. "Does the screen show it?" I ask.

Shawn nods, "A pretty strong one, actually."

It's nice to know the new epidural is working— at least for now. I am thankful that one thing, out of many, is going right.

"Here," Mom says as she slams the bag of potassium in Amy's hand. "Do you need me to hook it up, too?"

Amy smiles, "I have it under control. Thank you."

In my ignorant mind, I once believed that liquid hell was magnesium, until I met Stadol. After Stadol, I was convinced that Pitocin was the worst thing that would be pumping through my veins.

I was wrong. Liquid hell is, and always will be, potassium.

"It can't flow in with the others," Amy explains. "I need to make a new entrance point in your forearm."

Working as quickly as possible, she cleans my arm and shoves a needle into the skin. Holding the bag of potassium in the air, she squeezes it, forcing the contents into my body.

Ever light your arm on fire from the inside, Amy? No?

It's excruciating. If someone were to hand me a rusty saw in this moment, I would start to cut my arm off. I cry out in pain, but there is nothing that can be done to help me. I need the potassium, or I will die— plain and simple.

Shawn sits helplessly at my head, allowing me to burrow my face into his chest. I clench his shirt between my teeth, and cry in agony. I am so close to giving up; to losing this fight. I wish for it to end. I need this to be over.

I think about all the women who had shared their beautiful birth stories with me during my pregnancy and I'm insanely jealous. I feel like I got duped. This has been pure hell, and it's nowhere near over.

After two bags of potassium and the most painful thirty minutes of my life, my levels have stabilized. The epidural is working well, and my baby and I are out of immediate danger. I crave sleep; we all do. So after a cervix check with the doctor, I slowly allow my eyes to close and hope tomorrow will be a better day.

Day Three

I wake up to immense pressure in my bottom. It's like an elephant is sitting on my uterus while a watermelon is trying to push its way out.

Shawn and Mom are fast asleep on the other side of the room. I hesitate; unsure of whether waking them is the right thing to do. The pain quickly persuades me.

"Something hurts," I try to explain. "Is something wrong?"

I turn to my right and see a new nurse in Amy's seat. They must've switched shifts again while I was passed out. It didn't surprise me that I haven't noticed. Between the drugs and the extreme exhaustion, I was pretty much incoherent. I must've had my cervix checked a few times during the night, as well, but I can't remember.

A new resident walks through the doors. "How are things going in here?" she asks while applying her gloves.

"I have a lot of pressure down there," I explain, pointing to my vagina. I want to make sure she doesn't get confused on the location.

She lifts the sheet and checks my cervix. After only a few moments, she removes her fingers and greets me with a smile. "Congratulations, you're fully dilated and ready to push. I'll let your doctor know, and he should be in shortly."

Finally! The end is near. I search the room for a clock but can't locate it. I'm not sure what day it is, let alone the time. But, none of it matters; it'll all be over soon.

My new nurse, Jackie, pulls the stirrups from the side of the bed and a light from out of the closet. Another nurse wheels a bassinet into the far corner, along with a table filled with metal instruments that she places by my feet.

"Let's practice some pushing," Jackie explains. "Put your legs up in the stirrups. When you feel a contraction coming, I want you to bear down like you're having a bowel movement."

Bowel movement? No, that's not happening. I didn't get to take the birthing classes I wanted, but I am positive I'm not going to be pooping on this bed. Surely she must be mistaken.

I push with my vaginal muscles.

"Nope, that's not doing anything," she says.

How could she possibly know that? Is she inside my uterus? I wait for another contraction and push again.

"Nope. Nothing is happening, Ryan. You need to push in your butt," she instructs.

For some reason I always thought this phase would be quick. That once you make it to that point, it will only take a few pushes and the baby plops out into the doctor's hands.

Well, for me, that's not the case. I push with Jackie for almost two hours with very little progress. I can see the concern in her face as exhaustion weighs heavy on all of our bodies.

The doctor finally makes an appearance. It is the second time we have seen him during my pregnancy, and he definitely isn't our favorite.

Shawn and I silently exchange our disappointment. This is not who we hoped would be delivering our baby, but there isn't much we can do about it now.

"I'm going to put a vacuum extractor on your baby's head. It's obvious you need some help," the doctor states before he even offers a greeting.

No hello? And, was that an insult? This is my first time ever doing this, cut me some slack. But, he delivers babies all the time. Maybe, he's right? Maybe I do need help.

As scary as a vacuum or forceps may be, at this point, I don't care. I just want to be done. I am physically, emotionally, and spiritually exhausted.

"Ok," I agree to his decision even though my gut is telling me otherwise.

He instructs me to push, so I do. I stare in the lens of his glasses, hoping to be able to see Blake's head in the reflection— but I can't see anything. It would be encouraging to know if I'm making progress.

I should've opted for the mirror.

"I need to cut you," he says.

Before I can even resist, I see the scalpel slice in to my skin.

An episiotomy. I had never talked about it with the other OB's in the practice and I didn't really have a stance on it. However, I expected to be able to make a choice. Apparently, it is his choice to make, whether I agree or not.

Luckily, I can't feel the scalpel slice my skin, and within seconds, it's over.

"The pressure from the baby on your vagina will make you numb down there," Jackie explains. "It does seem like your epidural has worn off again, though," she adds.

Again? It has to be something I'm doing.

"Let's try another push," he commands.

With both his feet on the edge of my bed, and his hands wrapped around the vacuum, he leans back. I don't understand how he doesn't break my child's neck with the sheer amount of force he's using.

I push with all I have.

"Good. Keep going!"

[47]

Keep going? Does this man not know that I'm running on empty? I have no more left to give. I'm out. My body is caving on me. I cannot do it.

"Ryan, listen to me, two more pushes and you'll have a baby. Now, let's go!" he yells.

With Shawn on one side and Mom on the other, I swallow a breath of air and push with any ounce of fight I have left. The Doctor pulls, and I can feel her head slide out.

"Ok, stop pushing," he explains while suctioning fluid from her mouth. "She's face up, that's what made it hard to get her out. One more big push and you will have your baby."

The pain is indescribable. I want to get away from it, but there is nowhere to go, so I cry instead. The tears offer no relief from the burning ring of hell that is encompassing my entire vagina. Childbirth feels nothing like I imagined; it's so much worse.

"I cannot do it. It hurts so bad. Please, help me!"

I welcome death at the moment. I want to be anywhere else but here. I plead with Shawn. I beg him to help me; to get her out; to end this.

He stares in to my eyes. "One more, babe. Just one more, and then it's all over."

I have to do this, there is no other choice. I suck in a breath and scream it out, pushing with borrowed strength. Her shoulders emerge, followed by her back, hips and legs. Relief is instantaneous, and euphoria follows.

"She's here! She's beautiful!" Mom yells.

The doctor lays her on my chest for just a moment before the nurses sweep her away. Her tiny body is lifeless and her skin is blue instead of the pale pink everyone explains.

"She's not breathing," I hear one of them exclaim as she rubs her with a blanket.

"She's breathing, just not well," another corrects her.

As the nurses work to stabilize Blake, I deal with delivering the placenta. The OB massages my abdomen to stimulate contractions. It's awful. I want to be left alone, and the sheer annoyingness of being touched at this moment is driving me bonkers. I consider lifting my foot from the stirrup and handing him a swift kick to the head, but I resist. Even if I wanted to, I don't have the strength left to follow through.

Please leave me alone. I want to sleep and eat and hold my child. I want you—Dr. No name—to get the hell out of my room.

After what feels like forever, the placenta drops into the bowl and is swept out of the room. While I stare at the nurses who are struggling to steady Blake's breathing, he sews the wound *he* created only a short while ago.

Before my mouth can form any words, the nurses whisk my baby out of the room devoid of any explanation.

"Go with them," I insist to Shawn.

He hesitates. "What about you?"

"I'll stay with her," Mom promises. "Blake needs someone, too."

He drops my hand reluctantly and jogs to catch up to our daughter. It's killing me that I can't move from this bed. I can barely hold my head up and speak. I watch the door to the hallway close and wonder if Blake will be ok.

For a while, the nurses work to clean my battered body and I doze in and out, thinking about my baby.

"You'll need to stay on the magnesium until your blood pressure drops," Jackie explains. "Your potassium levels look much better, though."

I place a hand on my stomach, expecting to feel my baby's tiny kicks and punches. But, my finger sinks into the flab as I poke it. I'm finding it hard to grasp. We are now two separate beings, I am no longer growing a human in my body, and it's bittersweet. She is so vulnerable in this scary world.

What if delivering her is the thing that kills her? What if I failed at the one thing women are supposed to be able to do? My body is supposed to keep her safe, and I had to bring her out too soon.

I begin to weep. "When can I see her?" I beg.

[49]

The nurse shakes her head, "Not until you're stable. You're in no shape to get out of bed, plus you're still hooked up to lots of equipment. Perhaps in a few hours once we get you into your recovery room."

I don't like this nurse, either. How can you deny me from seeing my baby?

Shawn returns about an hour later. It was the longest hour of my life.

"Is she ok?" I ask.

"She's ok. Her breathing is slow and she's a little lethargic. They say it's from the magnesium and being premature. They want to keep her in the NICU a few days."

I'm worried. No one can prepare you for the sheer volume of fear that comes along with being a mother. It's never ending, and overwhelming. However, I try to relax. I know that the sooner I get into recovery, the sooner I can see her.

"Would you like some breakfast?" a woman bellows from the doorway.

Is this even a question?

"Considering I haven't eaten in about three days, and I'm dying of thirst. Yeah, breakfast would be swell."

Shawn elbows me, but I'm in no mood to deal with a chipper food delivery chick right now. However, I throw her a smile. If there's one thing I learned from years of waitressing, it's that you don't piss off the people that handle your food.

I place an order and throw my hair into a messy bun. I struggle to push myself into a seated position, and then immediately regret it when a pool of blood rushes from my vagina. An endless ache pulsates down below, and I lift the sheet to notice the mess that has soaked into the bed pad.

The nurse peeks over. "Let me change that and get you set up with something a little better."

She hands me a pair of stockings, a giant sanitary pad, and an ice pack. The ice is like heaven, and immediately offers relief from the throbbing but very little in absorbency. The nurse places a dry pad under me to catch the contents that continue to exit my uterus with even the slightest movement.

My breakfast arrives in the middle of cleaning up. I work to pull the stockings over my legs without getting out of the bed; afraid that my legs won't be able to hold the weight. After I have the ice and a pad on my wound, I cover myself with a warmed blanket and pull the food tray over to me.

The apple juice is my first victim. It's been over forty hours since I've had anything to eat or drink, and I'm about to ingest pure heaven. The cool wet liquid slides down my throat in one gulp. I should've savored it— allowed it to sit in my mouth for just a little while, but I couldn't resist. From there, I move on to my bottle of water— which I drink half of in just three swallows. Once my thirst is finally quenched, I devour my scrambled eggs and toast. It is, by far, the best meal I've eaten in my entire life.

Upon finishing, a nurse comes through the door with a wheelchair.

"Ready to move to recovery?" she asks.

I nod my head, knowing that I will be able to see my baby soon. Shawn cups his arms under me and easily lifts me from the bed to the chair. My tower of IV bags skates on the floor behind me as the nurse wheels it down the hall. I glance back with nostalgia at the room in which I delivered our daughter.

"We are out of beds in the labor & delivery unit, so we are putting you over in the geriatric wing. It's good though, because it's closer to the NICU where your baby is," she explains.

I want to respond, but I'm having trouble formulating the words. Exhaustion is winning the battle and my eyes go closed.

The jolt of the wheelchair wakes me. Shawn lifts me to the bed. I cover with a blanket and feel the river of fluid leak out with every position shift. I know I need to be changed, but I'm too tired to deal with the process.

"Let us know when you urinate, ok? We need to measure it. Also, if you have a bowel movement, just take note of it. If you need anything else, you can push the button."

She meanders toward the door while filling in my chart.
"When can I see my baby?" I inquire.

[51]

"Let me check with the NICU on visiting hours and get back to you," the nurse responds before leaving the room.

Visiting hours? You mean I can only see my baby at certain times? How is that even a real thing?

An hour later, while waiting for the nurse to return, I have an intense urge to urinate. I stand up with Mom's help, and shuffle to the bathroom in slow motion. Every step is torture on my battered body. I turn the corner, barely making it to the toilet seat and reaching for the red string on the way down.

"Mo---"

I wake up to Mom's arms struggling to lift me off the floor. I gather what strength I have left to get back on my feet.

"Come lie down," Mom instructs. "You passed out. I shouldn't have let you walk yet. You weren't ready."

The room spins as I lie back on the bed. The nurse tightens the cuff around my arm and pushes the button on the machine.

"75 over 65. Your blood pressure is too low. I'm gonna stop the magnesium now and call your doctor. You need to lie here until I come back. No getting out of bed."

"I want to see my baby," I cry.

Shawn hands me his phone after returning from his third trip to the NICU. My parents, brother, and two friends have already visited, and they have all gotten to meet Blake. I, unfortunately, have not. It's eating me alive how badly I want to hold her; to try to nurse her; to smell her hair and hold her hand.

I flip through the pictures as tears stream down my face. Her little eyes searching the room for me. Wondering where her mommy is. There are tubes sticking out of her and connecting to all of the machines that keep her body working. It's torturous to look at, and yet I can't stop.

She needs me and I'm not there.

I feel like a failure. It's my fault she's in there, because my body couldn't sustain the pregnancy. I can't take this anymore. I need to do something.

After begging the nurse for a breast pump, I place the phalange over my breast and extract the colostrum that is dripping from it. I don't know how long it will be until I get to nurse Blake, so I want to make sure she is getting these drops of liquid gold. Shawn walks the bottle down to the NICU once I'm finished—I'm envious of his fourth trip.

The nurse finally arrives a few hours later.

"Visiting hours in the NICU are over in 30 minutes. If you want to see your baby, you better get going."

I want to punch her.

You wasted 2 hours of time doing who knows what, that I could've spent with my daughter?

I'm too exhausted to lift my arm. She's lucky.

"Get me a wheelchair," I demand. "I am going to see my baby."

I scrub my hands and stare through the window at the tiny infants that fill the room. Shawn opens the door and pushes me through. I stare at each newborn as we pass. Tubes and wires attached to tiny bellies and mouths. Some are in incubators, and no bigger than Shawn's hand. Parents stand beside their cribs and whisper sweet words to their children, keeping faith in their journey while being unable to control it.

With every blue hat I pass, I know it's not Blake.

Finally, my chair comes to rest at the second to last bed on the left. In front of me, the most beautiful baby girl sleeps. Her eyes are closed, and her tiny head is covered with a pink hat. On her chest, there are multiple wires tracking her vitals. However, unlike how I imagined, there are no tubes helping her breathe. I hesitantly reach out to touch her hand, worried I might hurt her. Secretly, I hope she knows it's me.

"Hi, baby. My little angel," I whisper.

Tears fall down my cheeks and stain the blanket covering my lap.

"Would you like to hold her?" the nurse asks.

Fear and uncertainty overwhelm my body.

[53]

I have never held a baby in my life, and now I am going to be responsible for one so fragile? I am terrified.

"Can Shawn hold her first?" I ask, trying to buy myself some more time.

"Absolutely!"

The nurse wraps Blake in a blanket and hands her to Shawn. He sits in the rocking chair next to her crib, careful not to tug on any of the wires connected to her tiny body. I knew I loved this man, but seeing him hold our daughter makes me love him even more. It is pure bliss.

After a few minutes of watching them exchange glances, I am ready.

Shawn hands her to me, and I cup her head safely in my left elbow. Her mouth opens and she lets out a tiny whimper.

"Is she ok?" I ask frantically.

"She's perfectly fine," the nurse assures.

Adrenaline slows and exhaustion begins to take over. My arms shake and I quickly hand her back to Shawn.

"I can't," I cry. "My arms are too weak; I'll drop her."

The guilt eats me alive as I stare at my daughter being lifted off my lap. She needs me, and I failed her. I want to nurse her; to hold her; to smell her head—that fresh baby smell you read about in books—but I can't. I close my eyes and listen to the update from the nurse while Shawn changes her diaper. Moments later, I am awoken by them pulling the bottle of colostrum from my hand.

"Would you like me to feed her this?" the nurse asks.

I nod my head with what little energy I have left and then allow my eyes to close again. The day is over and I can't fight the fatigue anymore. I fall asleep in the wheelchair to the sound of Blake's cries.

Day Four

I awaken to the sun burning my face. The last few days feel like a dream, and it's not until I touch my stomach that reality sets in. Frantically, I search the room for Shawn who is resting in the chair beside me.

"How is she?" I ask, waking him from his slumber.

Shawn rubs his eyes and leans forward, placing his hand on mine. "She's doing fine. Get yourself around and I'll take you over," he explains.

He helps me to the bathroom, and after washing my face, I stare at my body in the mirror. It's battered and bruised from the last few days. My eyes are sunken and bloodshot, and my hair is disheveled in a messy bun above my ear.

As I reach in the sink to wash my hands, I notice the bruises—bruises from needles that are still being jabbed into them every few hours to draw blood and check my levels.

I take a seat on the toilet. A throbbing ache radiates through my bottom. I peek through my legs and notice the water in the bowl has been stained red. I pull the string on the wall to call the nurse, paranoid that I'm hemorrhaging.

She arrives swiftly. "Is everything ok?" she asks.

I open my legs and point to the bowl.

"It seems a little dark, but bleeding after delivery is very normal. Let's keep an eye on it for the next few hours to make sure everything is ok. How are you feeling besides that?"

"I feel better today. A little weak yet. Actually, it feels like I ran a marathon," I explain.

The nurse chuckles. "You did run a marathon, Hun. There ain't nothing easy about what you did. You can expect to be sore for a while."

Upon wiping, I notice dried blood on my inner thighs. "Do you think I could take a shower?" I inquire. "I feel disgusting."

I remember my friends telling me that the first shower after delivery is heaven. I need to bathe; besides seeing my daughter, washing off the horrors of the past few days is at the top of my to-do list.

"I'm sorry, but I don't know where to even find you a shower."

You can't find me a shower? This is a hospital, there has to be a million showers. Not one of these rooms has an available shower I can wash up in?

I force a smile as the nurse and I part ways and she leaves to help another patient. Sulking back to the bed I'm unable to hide the disappointment.

"What's wrong, babe?" Shawn asks.

"They won't let me shower," I whine.

He walks over to the suitcase and grabs a washcloth and soap. Leading me into the bathroom, he turns on the hot water.

"I'll wash you," he states.

I'm embarrassed—I know I look horrible, and I'm sure my odor is pungent, but Shawn is insisting. I take a seat on the toilet. The warm washcloth coasts down my arms and back, and the tension starts to fade. Feeling awkward, I tug on the stockings that are holding my pad in place; I can feel blood escaping my uterus with every shift of my body and I'm worried it will leak down my thigh. I pull down the gown, covering my bottom, making sure his eyes don't catch anything I don't want him to see.

[56]

"Is it ok if I do your legs?" he asks, sensing my hesitation.

I nod. As uncomfortable as I am, he is the opposite. I'm amazed at his commitment to me, and I allow him to wash the rest of my available skin before escorting him out of the room.

After dumping cups of warm water onto my vagina and allowing them to fall into the toilet, I dry myself with the towel. Yanking the hair tie from my bun, the smell of sweat hits me like a freight train. It's held stiff by grease, and I want to cry. I've never felt so disgusting in my life. Bending over the sink, I struggle to wash my hair. After a failed attempt, I flip it onto my head, and exit the bathroom. Although I'm not clean, I feel better.

I'm still weak on my legs and standing this long has made me shaky, so I take a seat in the wheelchair and allow Shawn to push me to the NICU. Blake is off the machines and lying in her crib wrapped in a blanket when we arrive.

"She's doing very well. She lost quite a bit of weight, so we've been trying to feed her often. Would you like to try?" the nurse asks.

I begin to open my gown as she hands me a bottle of formula. I glance over to the side table where my bottle of pumped colostrum remains, untouched from the night before. Anger boils in my blood, knowing that they didn't give her the one thing she needs the most.

"Why didn't you give her my colostrum? I'm going to breastfeed," I scold.

"Yes, well, since she was losing weight, and your milk didn't come in yet, we needed to supplement with formula. The colostrum wouldn't have been enough to satisfy her," she explains, shutting me down.

I am livid, but I have confidence that these nurses know what they are doing, so I seal my lips. I accept the bottle of formula and prepare to feed it to my hungry baby.

"Just keep pumping. Once your milk comes in, we can try to transition her over to nursing."

I nod my head as Shawn places Blake in my arms. Her body is wrapped in a white blanket. Her little eyes open to the sound of my voice. She glances throughout the room without really focusing on

[57]

anyone or anything. I stick the bottle in her mouth, so unsure of what I'm doing. Petrified, I hope a nurse will hear my invisible cries for help and assist me.

Nope, no one cares. The two nurses in the room have moved on to babies who need assistance. Shawn is standing at the desk, looking over her paperwork from the night before, and I am truly alone.

My body trembles.

No, Ryan. You cannot have a panic attack now. Not when your daughter needs you. Get it together.

With a deep breath, I focus on Blake as she starts to suckle and soon stops. A nurse walks toward me.

"Just be sure to burp her after every ounce," she blurts out and then walks away.

Don't just leave me here. Please? That's all you're going to say? I don't know what to do!

I stare at Shawn, pleading for his help.

"You're fine, Babe. You're doing just fine," he says, calmly. "I can help you burp her then. Just hold the bottle in there until she latches onto it. You'll get it."

I am petrified. Knowing that I'm personally responsible for her health and safety, is the scariest hand I've ever been dealt. She's mine, and that information hasn't quite sunk in.

✳✳✳✳✳

It is now Friday evening and Blake and I are supposed to be discharged tomorrow, however my blood pressure has become unsteady again and the doctors are concerned.

Sleep has become impossible. Every few hours, a nurse comes in, jostles me awake with the blood pressure cuff, stabs a needle in my arm to draw blood, and pulls down my underwear to check the stitches.

As crazy as it sounds, I think I have gotten used to strangers poking around my vagina. My modesty was left outside of the ER doors that first night, and I'm convinced it won't return until I walk through those doors again. It is uncomfortable, but necessary because infection can kill me.

Every two hours, I pump milk for our daughter. Finally, I can measure it in ounces rather than drops. However, I still haven't gotten a chance to put Blake to my breast—an opportunity I am hoping will come soon.

✳✳✳✳✳

The next morning, the nurses wheel Blake into my room like room service.

"She's discharged from the NICU," they exclaim. "She can stay in here with you."

A smile engulfs my face. It is such a nice surprise to start my day. Shawn hands her to me, and I immediately know what to do.

I whip out my right boob faster than I've ever done before, and put her mouth up to it. Nothing happens. I expected her to latch on and everything would be cake. I had visions in my head of her nursing instantaneously; that it would be easy and flawless. Instead, she roots around, unsure of what my nipple is, or how it works. She can smell my milk, and is definitely interested, but hasn't got a clue.

I glance around the room, but the two nurses have already left. Pushing the red button on my bed, I wait another few minutes for a nurse to arrive.

"Could you help me?" I ask, motioning to my breast.

"Absolutely, Hun. Let me just get your bloodwork done and then we will try to get your baby to eat."

Finally, someone who supports my decision to breastfeed.

I elongate my arm and hardly feel the needle pierce the skin. My left arm and hand have been destroyed from all the IV's and blood draws up until now, and my right arm has become irritated. Soon they will have to take it from my leg.

I sit in silence while the blood fills the vial, daydreaming about when we can leave this place.

"Ok, now, let's try the cradle hold. Just hold her with one arm with her head in your elbow. Push on her chin with your thumb

[59]

to get her to open her mouth. Then, position her mouth over your areola."

Her mouth opens, and she closes it on my nipple. Immediately, she begins suckling. Her tiny mouth turns into a vacuum. It's a force of suction that no one can prepare you for and it takes me completely off guard. I fight every urge in my body to pull my nipple back out of her mouth and flee.

"Try to relax," the nurse explains. "Take a deep breath. Leave her nurse as long as she will like. It looks like she's latched on ok. I'll let you have some time. Ring the bell if you need me."

I smile through the pain, thanking her for the help. Then, I struggle to get comfortable. Once I get over the initial shock of the latch, I ease into the strange new feeling.

I stare at Blake, breathing in her scent. I feel like I have waited forever for this moment and yet it all went by so quickly. Twenty minutes later, she's asleep at my breast and I transition her to the crib next to me, as the nurse instructed me to do.

I watch her chest rise and fall with each breath and realize that it isn't just Shawn and I anymore—we are responsible for this tiny human, and what a journey it is going to be.

Day Five

The morning light blasts through the window onto Blake's crib. Neither Shawn nor I got much sleep, but it's expected with a newborn. On my morning trip to the bathroom, I am still bleeding quite heavily and it's quite worrisome. I call the nurse in to see the amount of blood on my pad, but she assures me it's normal and I am simply overreacting.

"The doctor will be in soon to discharge you," she explains. "This is all the normal process of healing. Try not to worry."

My breasts are engorged, so I pump as Blake sleeps. Shawn packs our suitcase while we wait for the doctor to arrive.

✶✶✶✶✶

"I'm keeping you another day," the OB explains from the edge of my bed. "Your blood pressure's just not where I want it to be and we are still watching your potassium. Also, your daughter has jaundice. She will need to go in the nursery full-time to be under the light."

I hug Blake in my arms, refusing to let go. "Is it something I should be worried about?"

The doctor laughs. "No. It's very common. It'll subside in a few days. Formula feeding is recommended. I'm not sure which feeding method you are using currently."

"Well, I'm trying to breastfeed, but she's had formula."

I stare at the tiny baby in my arms, all six pounds of her. I can see her skin has a slightly yellow hue.

"The nurse will be in to get her soon. If you have any questions, she will be able to answer them. I'll check in with you later."

I turn to Shawn, defeated. "I just got her and they are taking her away again." Tears flow down my cheeks as Blake begins to whimper. "We are never getting out of here, are we?"

He wraps his arms around us, and takes a seat on the bed. "One step at a time."

✳✳✳✳✳

Blake lies under the blue light for most of the day. I pump and send my milk down, and they choose to supplement with formula. Every two hours, I hook the suction cup to my nipples and listen to the motor groan with each pump. Tiny sprays of milk come out, but with every ounce that fills the bottle, I know it will probably never see my daughter's stomach.

Pacing the floors of the hall, I mope. I want to hold my baby. I want her to drink the milk I am pumping. I want to begin forming a bond with her, but I'm starting to feel disconnected and depressed.

I visit her every hour, and finally, sometime in the afternoon, they let me hold her again. I stare at her lying under the blue light with cloth covering her eyes.

"Don't worry about the cuts on her heels. Every few hours we have to take blood to check her bilirubin levels. No big deal," the nurse explains while she peels the bandage back to show us.

My heart aches. I finally understand the turmoil of being a mother. There is no amount of love that ever compares to the love I have for my child. I want to scoop her up and hold her close to my chest to assure her that momma is here; that everything is going to be ok. Instead, I'm helpless, standing beside her crib and watching her sleep under the light with only a diaper covering her yellow skin.

Tiny wisps of brown hair peek out from under her pink hat. The nurse switches off the light, removes the cover from her face and wraps her in a blanket. As she hands her to me, Blake opens her eyes.

It is absolute magic. She tries to look at me, but has trouble focusing. Her eyes are searching the room. They even roll back into her head a few times. I feel anxiety sliding up my body as uneasiness takes a hold of my stomach.

The nurse notices my change of energy and places her hand on my shoulder. "They can't see that great yet, so their eyes don't really focus. It'll come. It's completely normal."

A sigh of relief sneaks out as the panic begins to fade. Blake begins to fuss and root at her hands.

"She's hungry; would you like to feed her?"

I nod my head. The nurse hands me a bottle as I struggle to get my breast exposed through the gown.

"Isn't she on formula?" she asks.

I shake my head. "I've been pumping and bringing milk down for her. They told me that you would supplement with formula if I wasn't producing enough, but breastmilk is supposed to come first."

"Oh, well I have this bottle all ready for you. Do you want to just use it so it doesn't get wasted?"

I feel agitated. I know I want to breastfeed and that it is what's best for her, but it seems like I'm fighting a losing battle. The nurses continue to push for formula, and considering they are around babies all the time, I trust their advice.

I accept the bottle and feed it to her. I'll pump once I get back to the room to relieve my aching breasts. Now that I told the nurse, I'm confident she will be getting my milk during her feedings.

Blake finishes her formula and lets out a few good burps. I change her diaper and hand her back to the nurse who positions her on the table under the light. I sit with her for a bit longer and watch her sleep before heading back to the room to eat supper.

Tomorrow is Easter Sunday and day six of our hospital stay. Shawn and I are hopeful that we will finally get to take Blake home, but there's no telling what tomorrow may bring.

[63]

Home for the Holidays

"Her bilirubin levels are stable enough that you guys can get discharged today. You will need to bring her back tomorrow and probably the next day for blood work, though. I'm sending a UV blanket home with you. She will need to wear it most of the day. Your insurance will cover it."

We are thrilled. Finally, we get to take our baby home. I get to hold her for hours without anyone telling me I can't or wheeling her out of the room. I can refuse formula and breastfeed her when she is hungry. Diaper changes, naps, burps, and baths are all up to me, and I cannot wait.

"It feels weird," I say from the bathroom.

"What does?" Shawn yells from the bed.

"Wearing real clothes. I've been in that gown for a week."

I place a maxi pad in my underwear, and worry that it won't be enough to control the bleeding until we get home. Blake cries, and I can feel my milk let down, creating circles on my shirt. Quickly, I grab toilet paper and shove it in my bra, hoping it will be enough. The nurse notices the milk stains and offers me two breast pads from the hallway closet.

"I can't believe we are leaving," I say as we walk out of the hospital doors. The temperature is in the 40's and it's been raining all morning. I stare at our tiny baby and worry she will catch a chill.

"I'll throw this over the car seat," Shawn says as he unzips his coat. "It'll keep the rain off her. The fleece blanket should keep her warm enough. I'll pull the car around. You wait inside until I come back."

The nurse stays with me until Shawn returns. Blake sleeps in the car seat on the floor at my feet.

"Do you have any questions or concerns, Ryan? I know it can be scary going home. Especially after all you've been through."

My head shakes, "No. I'm just ready to get out of this place. No offense."

She giggles, "None taken. I don't blame you at all. You enjoy that little sweetheart."

Shawn's t-shirt is soaking wet as he runs through the rain into the lobby. Carrying Blake to the car he shields her with his coat. The nurse assists me to the door and waves goodbye after handing me over to Shawn.

I sit in the back on the way home, paranoid that Blake will need me. My bottom aches, and I should've sat on the pillow Shawn offered before we left. Listening to me whine in discomfort for most of the ride, he offers to pull over, but I refuse. At this point, I just want to be home.

When we finally arrive, it's surreal. Shawn carries the car seat and I lag behind with a vase of flowers.

"Welcome home, Blake," he says.

I blubber—an ugly cry mixes snot and tears around my face.

Damn hormones.

Pulling a tissue out of the box, I take a seat on the couch. Shawn unstraps Blake from her seat and hands her to me. For the first time in almost a week, I get to hold my baby without being watched or lectured. I get to snuggle and kiss her, endlessly. I can unapologetically stare at her for hours, studying every little inch of her face, engulfing myself in her perfection.

[66]

Shawn unloads the car before taking a seat next to me. Together, in silence, we relish in the moment of gratitude and awe, staring at our beautiful baby girl.

Ten minutes later she is awake and hungry. I offer my breast and she latches on, but almost immediately spits it out. I try again, but her cries quickly turn to anger. I switch to a different hold and then offer her the other breast, but nothing works.

"Get the bottle from the bag. I have some pumped milk on the side. See if she will drink that."

Shawn pours my—minuscule—two ounces of pumped milk into the bottle and I rub the nipple across her lips. Immediately, she latches and begins suckling.

Tears stream down my face. "She doesn't want my breast. She doesn't want me. I'm a failure! It's too late."

I know it's over— she is never going to nurse. I hand her to Shawn and retreat to the bedroom to pump my aching breasts. It was never in my plan to be a "pumping mom", but I'll do what I need to for her. Hopefully my body can keep up.

After she finishes, we cover her in the UV wrap and a fleece blanket. Shawn rocks her on his chest until she falls asleep and I sneak off to enjoy the first shower I've had in a week.

The warm water runs over my tired skin, washing all the pain and bitter memories away. I worry that the water will burn as it runs across my stitches, but it doesn't. My hair is begging for shampoo as I turn and wet it, the lingering scent of hospital sheets hits my nose and a bittersweet feeling emerges. I may never give birth again, and I wanted to get out of that hospital so badly, that I forgot to enjoy the moments.

A half-hour later, I'm clean and refreshed. I hurry back to the living room where Blake is sleeping on Shawn's chest. I'm jealous and feel left out. He winks at me, and encourages me to join him, but I decide to throw some laundry in the dryer and unpack our hospital bag instead.

We set up the bassinet next to our bed and put Blake in it after her next bottle. I stare at her for a long time before fatigue takes over and I drift off to sleep.

The night is long and interrupted. Shawn awakens every time I do, and feeds her the bottle while I pump my engorged breasts. Thankfully, I am able to remain one session ahead on my milk, so I don't have to supplement with formula. I'm pretty sure that we are walking zombies by morning, and I don't know how we are going to get through the day.

After getting up and around, we drive Blake back to the hospital for bloodwork. Negative thoughts engulf my mind, and I fret about the possibility of them wanting to admit her again.

The nurse wipes her foot with an alcohol pad before pricking her heel with a tiny needle. A few seconds pass before she emits a blood-curdling scream. It is heart wrenching, and I struggle to hold it together as I bounce her through the pain.

I don't know how to get her to stop. People are going to think I'm a horrible mother.

"Blake's levels are improving," the nurse explains. "She's not out of the woods yet, so I still need her to wear the light, and you'll have to come back again tomorrow."

"But, it's getting better?" Shawn asks.

"Yes," the nurse responds. "She should be fine within a few days. But, we just need to be sure before we remove the UV light completely."

Blake has settled and I place her back in the car seat, careful not to pinch her delicate skin while I hook the clasps. We schedule our appointment and exit the doors again.

I'm relieved, and wait on the bench with Blake while Shawn runs to get the car. The spring sun heats my body, quite a difference in weather from yesterday. I toss my sweater over Blake to protect her from the sun's rays.

Five minutes later, Shawn pulls the car around. I grab the car seat and carry it to meet him. There is a pillow waiting for me on the seat next to her, and my aching bottom is relieved to see it.

[68]

Once home, I stand up and feel something fall out of my vagina. I waddle to the bathroom and pull down my pants, slowly. Sitting in my underwear, is a blood clot the size of a plum. I pull a piece of toilet paper from the roll and scoop it up, examining it in my hand. Nauseated by it, and extremely worried, I allow it to fall into the toilet, but don't flush. Exiting the bathroom in a panic, I grab my phone and call the doctor.

"I think I'm hemorrhaging, or something!" I yell at the nurse. "This thing came out of me."

"Did you lift more than ten pounds?" she asks calmly.

"No. Wait, yes! Why?"

"It's just a blood clot. You overdid it and sometimes this happens. It's not uncommon, but you need to take it easy. Ok?"

I thank her and hang up, unsure about the seriousness of what happened.

How can that thing be normal? I don't think she understood how big it was!

The rest of the day, I'm in and out of the bathroom every 30 minutes to check for clots. Each trip yields different results. Sometimes, small clots stare at me from the toilet, other times it's simply a blood soaked pad. I refuse to hold Blake while standing, or lift her from the bassinet all day. Tears run down my cheeks from frustration. My body continues to fail over and over again and there's nothing I can do about it.

✶✶✶✶✶

The following day, we are back at the hospital for bloodwork. I hold her while they prick her heel, and once again she screams. I pray that her levels are good enough this time that we don't need to bring her back tomorrow because I'm not sure how much more I can take.

"Her levels look good. You don't need to do the UV light anymore. I would sit her in the sun in the window for about ten minutes twice a day if you can; it'll help speed things up. But, she should be fine. Here's a list of things to watch for."

We leave the hospital and head to the pediatrician for Blake's one week check-up. I am hopeful that she is gaining well and they won't push formula too hard.

Waiting in the back room for a while, Blake begins to shiver. The nurse instructed us to strip her down to her diaper, but then never came back. I wrap her naked body in a blanket and hold her in my arms, annoyed with the entire office.

"Ok, let's get her on the scale and check her out," a nurse busts through the door.

What? No apologies? No introductions? Time to find a new pediatrician.

Blake winces away from the cold metal of the scale and begins to cry as soon as Shawn lays her on it. My heart aches, again. This is absolute torture.

"Six pounds, four ounces," the doctor says. "What was her birthweight?"

"Six, six," I respond, quickly, hoping it will get her off the scale sooner.

"Ok, that's not bad. She's expected to lose some the first few days, and then she should start gaining. It says she was six pounds when she was discharged. So, she's back to gaining. Perfect. Is she nursing?" she asks without making eye contact.

I grab her off the scale without the doctor's permission, and press her against my body. "I'm pumping," I respond, defeated.

"Ok. I'll need you to take that blanket off."

I don't want to take her blanket off.

Reluctantly, I remove it and lie her down on the exam table. Her body retracts as soon as she hits the paper. Her arms flail and her eyes turn wide. My heart breaks into a million pieces, and the hatred for the doctor grows.

"Let's measure her length," she says. "Nineteen inches. She's really not a bad size for being premature," she explains while she measures her head. "Oh, big head. Poor momma," she laughs.

I don't find it funny. My vagina aches while I sit on the cold metal chair. Flashbacks of the delivery scream through my mind. Shawn places his hand on my shoulder, sensing my anxiety.

After a thorough exam, she hands Blake back to me and I zip her fleece pajamas over her cool skin. She is rooting for some milk, so I retrieve the bottle from the bag. It's been a busy morning and I haven't been able to pump yet to replenish, I know the empty bottle is not going to fill my little girl's belly.

We head to the car and I attempt to breastfeed, praying she will latch on. She screams when my nipple doesn't give her what she wants fast enough, but I have no choice but to try again. She latches, and I feel the milk let down. She suckles for a few minutes before falling asleep in my arms.

"I can't believe she did it!" I yell at Shawn. "She drank from my breast!"

Tears of joy fly down my cheeks and land on her head. I refuse to move while she naps. After twenty minutes of allowing her to dream suckle, I transfer her to the car seat and we head home.

Once there, I pump the milk from my other breast to prepare for our next feeding and attempt to throw a load of laundry in. I bend down to lift the clothes pile into the washer and feel a gush from my vagina. I run to the bathroom.

Yet again, another plum-sized clot stares at me from my underwear. Frustrated, I drop it in the toilet and take a seat on the couch to rest.

I guess I'll have to take it easy for a while yet—my body won't have it any other way.

Six Weeks

Six weeks pass and I can't believe our daughter is almost two months old; time flies and yet stands absolutely still. The plum-sized clots are still occurring quite regularly, but every time I call the OBGYN, they are convinced it's just my body's way of telling me to slow down. Today is my postpartum check-up and I am—per usual—incredibly anxious.

"So, how have you been feeling?" Doctor "overalls" asks with a cheesy grin.

I see you landed on a flannel shirt and jeans for your outfit choice today— professionalism is definitely high on your list, I see.

"I'm still bleeding quite a bit," I explain. "I'm also throwing pretty big clots once in a while. Is that normal?"

"Well, women can bleed for six weeks after delivery. Usually small clots, about the size of grapes, are normal in the early stages of bleeding."

"I'm throwing plum sized clots, multiple times per week. Also, I'm still bleeding like a heavy period."

He reads over my paperwork. "Vaginal delivery?"

"Yes," I respond.

"Any complications?"

"Preeclampsia. He used a vacuum, and I had an episiotomy. My baby was sent to the NICU. My potassium was low. I was in the hospital for a week," I ramble.

"Let's take a look," he cuts me off and motions me to lie back.

I slide down to the end of the table and place my legs in the stirrups. It doesn't matter how many times I do this, it never gets easier. He glances at my scar before putting a metal device into my vagina and cranking it open.

"Here's the issue," he says as he grabs a tool out of the drawer. "You have pieces of placenta stuck in your cervix."

He removes the pieces in only a few seconds.

"There. You're bleeding should calm down now," he explains.

I sit up while he continues talking; fixing the paper blanket that covers my lap.

"Why didn't you come in? We could've fixed this weeks ago. You're lucky you didn't get an infection."

Are you kidding me?

I explain to him how I had called on several occasions. He makes a note in my chart and then moves on to talk about birth control, refusing to acknowledge the fault in his office staff.

"What will you be using?"

"Condoms," I reply.

"Well, we have hormonal birth control options which are more reliable. Condoms can break."

I nod my head, "I don't respond well to hormonal birth control. We will be using condoms."

He hands me paperwork on other birth control options, including a hormone free IUD. I reluctantly accept so he exits the room.

"Once you're bleeding stops, you are cleared for your normal activities. Until then, I would stay away from sex."

[74]

With an awkward wink, he leaves the room. I schedule my yearly pap smear, and exit the office.

I head home and pump. My right breast expels one ounce, and I pray my left will yield more. Fifteen minutes later, I'm disappointed to see that it hasn't.

I know that it isn't going to be enough for Blake, and I prepare formula in a separate bottle. I don't want to stop breastfeeding. I dreamed about doing it for as long as Blake wanted to. I read about self-weaning and how beneficial it is for babies to nurse until they are at least two. But, my dreams are beginning to fade.

✶✶✶✶✶

At eight weeks postpartum, my breasts are only producing around an ounce total, and I decide to switch Blake to formula full-time. It's bittersweet. I thought I would have this amazing relationship with nursing; that we would form this bond and my breasts would produce enough milk to nourish her for at least the first year, but my body failed to do that.

She falls asleep on my lap while drinking her bottle, and I cry. I've failed to give her the one thing that should come naturally. I don't feel like a woman. I'm not sure why my body hasn't been able to keep up, but I hold all the blame. Depressed feelings hang on for weeks as I struggle with postpartum depression.

"I think I need to talk to someone," I state as I watch Shawn rock Blake to sleep. "I just feel—I don't know—."

He nods his head. "Why don't you go see Ruth again? She helped you before."

Ruth was my therapist from a few years back. She has helped me numerous times I've struggled with my anxiety, and I'm confident she will know how to help me with the depression. I pull her card from my wallet, dial her number, and make an appointment for the following week.

"So, what brings you in, Ryan? Trouble with your anxiety again?" Ruth asks as she welcomes me into her office and pulls the door closed.

"Baby blues," I say, defeated.

"You had a baby? That's wonderful! Congratulations!"

I thank her, while trying to hold it together.

"I see you're having trouble now. Do you want to talk about it?" she asks as she scribbles down notes on her pad.

"I failed," I wail. "I just can't do it. I'm a horrible mother! The one thing I was supposed to do, I couldn't. I'm still bleeding! My body hates me!"

"Oh my. That must be so stressful," Ruth says as she hands me a box of tissues. "What do you think you failed at?"

"Everything," I respond, curtly.

"I assure you, Ryan. You have not failed at everything. Is your daughter fed?"

"Yes," I respond.

"Dressed?"

"Yes."

"Does she have a bed, and a home, and a mother and father?"

What is your point?

"Yes," I force through clenched teeth.

"Well, I don't consider that failing. In fact, I think you're doing pretty damn well."

I disagree, but remain quiet.

"Ryan, listen to me: being a mother is—by far—the hardest job you will ever do in life. You will fail sometimes, but you will also achieve great things. You will question every single decision you ever make. You will worry about your children constantly, and that won't fade as the years pass. No one is perfect, and we just do our best. You have to remember that you are human."

[76]

"I understand that, but I couldn't breastfeed. I couldn't make something that all women should be able to do. What is wrong with me?" I interrupt.

"I'm not a lactation specialist, Ryan. But, perhaps it wasn't something you did wrong. Maybe it wasn't anything you could control. I was unable to nurse my oldest son because of complications during delivery. I was in recovery for so long, that my body was more focused on healing than on producing milk. Did you have a complicated delivery?"

I nod my head as thoughts fly through it.

Maybe it was the bleeding? That damn piece of placenta in my cervix ruined everything! It wasn't my fault that I couldn't breastfeed, it was the doctors'!

"Ryan? Would you like to share what's going on in your head?"

Ruth is incredible. I've been on this couch for ten minutes and she's figured out things I've been struggling with for months.

"Things are just making sense," I explain. "You solved my puzzle."

"Well, that's good. Do you think it'll help you feel better?"

"I'm not sure if it will, but it's a start."

We talk for a while longer about my delivery and life with Blake. She offers some tips to handle my depression and advises me to attend weekly sessions with her until I feel stable.

✳✳✳✳✳

Arriving home, Blake is awake in her swing while Shawn cooks dinner. I walk over to her and kneel down.

"Hi, baby girl," I whisper.

Blake's eyes sparkle and the most beautiful smile encompasses her face.

"Babe!" I exclaim.

"Her first smile!" Shawn cheers. "She really missed you. She loves her mommy, so much."

[77]

I lean in and kiss her on the forehead as tears fill my eyes and my vision turns blurry.

"Maybe I haven't failed everything."

The Next Five Years

Years go by so quickly when you become a mother. Chasing a child around really makes time fly.

We are so fulfilled by Blake. We know she is enough, and I got rid of all of her baby stuff as quickly as she outgrew it. We accepted that we were lucky; that we both made it through ok, and we were here. We weren't going to chance something happening to me if we decided to try for another. I couldn't stand the idea of Blake having to grow up without a mom.

My father got diagnosed with cancer in the summer of 2014, and it shook me to the core. As my siblings and I rallied around him, I sat and wondered how hard it would be for Blake when Shawn and I got old. She would be alone, and all the weight would fall on her shoulders. What would happen to her after we passed away?

I felt sad. I felt like Preeclampsia stole an opportunity that she should've been offered. This complication took that potential sibling from her, and it made me livid.

"I think she needs a sibling," I spit out in the middle of dinner.

"No way," Shawn objects. "It's way too risky. What if something happens?"

I know he's right, but I also know there are other ways to have a baby.

"Ok, but how about adoption?" I ask.

Shawn makes eyes at me as he refuses to talk about it in front of Blake who is all ears.

"What's adoption, Mommy?" she asks.

"Now you did it," Shawn snarls.

"Nothing, sweetie. Adult stuff that Daddy and I need to talk about privately."

I change the subject to the fall leaves outside, and drop my silverware onto my plate. I've lost my appetite for now.

A pregnancy for me is far too risky, but there is just something that's missing and I need to find it.

For weeks, I search the internet for options. The price to pay a surrogate is out of our range, and the process of harvesting my eggs isn't something I'm on board with. Crossing it off the list, I look into adoption agencies—both national and international.

"It says here it's about 30 grand to adopt a baby," I yell from the bedroom.

"Yeah?" Shawn asks as he walks toward me.

"Yeah, and it can take years."

As Shawn takes a seat on the bed, I skim the article on the computer screen.

"This birth mother changed her mind after the baby had already gone home with the adoptive parents. She got the baby back! Can you imagine? What if that happened to us? I would be devastated!" I yell.

"Ok, well, we aren't doing adoption," Shawn demands as he pretends to cross it off the list. "What's our next option?"

A friend of mine had talked about doing foster-to-adopt after she had a complicated pregnancy. She wanted more kids, but physically couldn't put her body through it again. After researching private adoption, she decided to look into other options, and landed on the foster-to-adopt program.

[80]

From what she explained, it only cost a couple thousand dollars from start to finish. You could adopt any age, gender, and ethnicity. You would foster them for a while, and once their parents' rights were terminated, you would have the opportunity to permanently adopt.

"Can we get a baby, though?" Shawn asks. "I'm not comfortable with an older kid."

"I'm not sure. Becky said it was all ages," I say, staring at the computer screen.

I type **foster to adopt in Pennsylvania** in the search bar, and click on the top link.

Shawn answers a work call and I sit on the bed scrolling through their "available" children. The feeling of shopping for a child is strange, but I continue on. A thirteen year old, red-haired girl catches my attention, and I read her profile. She is adorable. She likes to read and play piano and has been in foster care—shuffled from family to family—for most of her life. My heart aches for her, and I wonder what it would be like to invite a teenage foster girl into our home.

Blake is now five years old, and I have to think about how this would affect her. She is such a timid kid and extremely sensitive. She doesn't talk to strangers, or join in with children playing at the park. She's always been more of distant observer. Questions begin to flood my mind. What if she grows attached? What if the adoption doesn't work and they have to go back? What if her parents come looking for her and we are in danger?

I shut the computer, and cross foster-to-adopt from my list. A tear races down my face as my heart breaks for the children with no homes. It takes an amazing person to be a foster parent, and I wish I was that person, but I'm not.

My list is dwindling. I have two viable options left, neither of which I like. One is to risk a second pregnancy, and the other is to not even try.

I join Shawn in the living room as he finishes his call and take a seat on his lap. "What are we going to do?"

He strokes my hair and kisses my forehead. "We go talk to some doctors," he whispers, "and then we make a decision."

[81]

Research has become my middle name, and it is a plan I can get on board with.

The next morning, I call a maternal-fetal specialist and schedule an appointment. They are specialists in things like Preeclampsia, and should be able to give us realistic expectations for a subsequent pregnancy. Two weeks later, we are on our way to her office.

"So, what brings you in?" she asks from behind her desk.

I lean forward to hand her my records. "I had Preeclampsia in my first pregnancy, and I'm looking for some statistics on my chances of getting it again. We really want to try for another baby, but are terrified."

Shawn and I sit in silence while Blake colors at the table next to us. Ten minutes pass while the doctor looks over every piece of paper in my file.

"Do you have history of Preeclampsia? Did your mother have it?"

"No," I respond.

"Aunts, sisters, grandmothers?" she asks.

"I don't think so," I answer.

"Hmm, ok."

I lean back on the chair and fold my hands on my lap. Blake walks over with a picture.

"This is for you, Mommy," she says in her adorable little voice.

The doctor interrupts, "Ok, well, the problem with Preeclampsia is that we have no idea what causes it. We don't know why some women get it and some don't. All we know is that it's an issue with the placenta, and that the only cure is delivery."

We nod our heads, "Right."

Tell me something I don't know.

"Well, you have no family history. No hypertension, no heart problems. You're not overweight—you're in good shape. I feel like it's a fluke. Now, because you had it, you are already considered high risk in any subsequent pregnancy. Your chance of getting it again is a lot higher than someone who's never had it."

She pauses to read the paper, and then asks, "When did you deliver?"

"36 weeks," I say.

"Ok, that's not too bad. Let me see your levels here ... and, your protein. Blood pressure," she talks to herself.

"Hmm, in my opinion? I think you probably have about a 30-40% chance of getting it again. Some women get it worse and earlier, some get it less severe and later. And, a few don't get it at all. There is absolutely no way to predict which one you will be."

I let out a deep sigh.

"I would recommend going into a pregnancy as prepared as possible. Stress is not a good thing, so you have to find a way to not be afraid. Also, you should start your prenatal vitamins and a daily blood thinner. Eat healthy, and exercise regularly. It should help."

She stands and reaches out to shake my hand. "Any more questions?"

"No," I respond. "Thank you."

I motion to Blake that it's time to go and she cleans up, packing the crayons neatly back into the box. Shawn opens the door and we walk to the car in silence. Once the doors close, he loses it.

"Forty percent chance of losing you or the baby? That's not a risk I'm willing to take. We have Blake," he says, fighting tears, "let's count our blessings and move on. I cannot watch you go through that again. I can't lose you."

I wrap my fingers around his and force out an encouraging smile. "I understand." I feel the dream of another baby slipping out of my grasp, and there isn't a damn thing I can do about it.

✳✳✳✳✳

About six months pass, but I have never given up on my future baby. Being a stay-at-home mom, I spend a good portion of time researching Preeclampsia. I read every article I can get my hands on. Web articles, clinical trials, women's testimonials, multiple blogs and online groups litter my house.

I have all the information I can to try and figure things out; to form some sort of solution to this fear.

A lot of studies seem to have one common belief: that Preeclampsia is a result of the mother's immune system rejecting the embryo. It attacks the placenta as its forming and damages it, causing it to malfunction. The blood flow is compromised, and eventually it leads to Preeclampsia. Based on the amount of damage caused, the Preeclampsia will show its severity at different weeks in the pregnancy.

Ok, it makes sense. My body saw Blake as an intruder or foreign body, so it attacked her, damaging the placenta. They caught the signs of damage on the twelve week blood work but couldn't find a way to fix it, so they prescribed the blood thinner to help with the blood flow. Once the medicine stopped, the blood thickened back up, put more pressure on the veins, and my blood pressure elevated to dangerous levels.

I understand the process. Now, I need to figure out how to prevent it.

So, I do more research.

Our immune system is basically an army. Its main goal is to protect us from bacteria and viruses that try to destroy us. If my body is seeing the embryo as a threat, how can I change that?

I have an idea: a few days ago on a cooking show, the chef was allergic to shrimp. He said he got tired of wearing gloves all the time when he cooked, so one day he just decided to deal with it. His hands swelled up, his arms were covered in hives, and he was out of work for a few days.

But, instead of quitting, he did it again. The same thing happened and his body responded with an overreaction. However, this time it regressed quicker and he was back to work the next day. He continued working with the shrimp, and his body gave less of a reaction each time until it realized that the shrimp wasn't a threat.

Eventually, his allergy subsided.

Is this reality? Who knows- It's on television.

So, I did what any sane human would do—I looked it up on the internet.

Can you be allergic to sperm/semen?

I can't believe the answers that pop up. Women who swear they have reactions to their partner's semen. The worst instances were their vaginas swelling or their throats closing up after swallowing. I am shocked at some of the stories they are sharing with complete strangers, but I'm thrilled with the information.

What if Preeclampsia really was the result of an immune response; almost like an allergy? What if I could get my body "used" to my husband's "genetic makeup" before I got pregnant again. Would it help?

I don't take hormonal birth control for many reasons, so we have relied on condoms and the withdrawal method for many years after Blake. It has been almost six years since he "released" inside me, and I wonder how my vagina would respond.

Even if I can get on board with this idea, I need to be sure I won't get pregnant.

A friend of mine has used NFP (Natural family planning) as birth control for many years. It involves tracking your cycle and abstaining from sex during your fertile window. After you ovulate—and the egg dies—until your period, you have zero chance of getting pregnant (as long as you don't ovulate twice in one cycle). So, if done correctly, you can have sex with no form of birth control.

Essentially, I can follow the chef's advice and allow my body to overcome its immune reaction to my husband's sperm without the chance of getting pregnant.

I have a fleeting moment of worry before I realize one thing: having sex without a condom is every man's dream, so convincing Shawn should be a relatively easy task.

Putting it to the Test

"How about three months?" I ask Shawn.

He looks hesitant, but isn't going to argue against unprotected sex. "Fine, three months. But, you are one-hundred percent sure you can't get pregnant with this, right?"

I nod my head. "Do you want me to show you the paperwork about this method again? Explain to you, in detail, the female reproductive system?"

"No," he responds while I barely finish my question. "I don't want to hear about all that stuff. I trust you. I'm just not ready yet for you to be pregnant. Not until I'm sure."

"I know, babe. I'm sure about this. Just trust me," I beg.

✳✳✳✳✳

The first time we have sex, my vagina burns like fire after the semen hits it. For days, I feel like I shoved a tampon made of sandpaper inside me and ripped it out. My abdomen is also tender and feels full every time I go from a standing to sitting position. It's torturous and I consider calling the gynecologist because I'm convinced that I have some sort of infection. To ease the pain, I take a warm bath every night and pray it's not Shawn's semen that my body is overreacting to.

[87]

In a few days, the pain subsides and we try again. A few hours after, it yields similar results. I cry in the bathtub, wondering if my body will ever get used to him. I know that if it doesn't, my chances of pregnancy are slim to none.

Another week passes and my period is a welcomed escape— giving my body a few days to recuperate. The sight of a bloody pad validates my research that the NFP method has worked, and Shawn has nothing to worry about. After the cramps and achiness from menses subside, everything is back to normal, and I'm excited to try again.

During month two, my body's reaction is similar, but has decreased in intensity. I am shocked that I can notice a difference and toss it up to a fluke occurrence. I decide to increase the frequency of our sexual encounters, hoping to see some sort of reaction. Even though it is irritated, it's not nearly as bad as the month prior. I'm trying to hold back my premature excitement, but perhaps this experiment will hold merit.

By month three, we are falling in love with NFP. We can have sex most of the time without having to remember a condom, and my body is now showing very little reaction to Shawn's semen. Who knows if it's coincidental, or if my theory is working, but I decide to share with Shawn what I have discovered.

"I think it'll be ok," I spit out while lying in bed. "I think my body will allow the baby to form without attacking it. We were so new before. We used condoms up until we got pregnant with Blake. It never had a chance to get used to the proteins, and it felt threatened."

Shawn stares at me like I have three heads.

"Don't look at me like that," I scold. "I've been researching this for months. It makes sense. I'm not saying it's foolproof and that I won't get Preeclampsia again, but I think it's definitely a good sign."

He smiles with fear. "It does make sense, but what if..."

"We will cross that bridge if it comes," I cut him off. "I can't not have another one. I cry whenever I think about it. And, all the other options just aren't going to work."

[88]

"We are finding a new doctor," he demands. "And, you will buy a blood pressure monitor, too. And— and ..."

I nod my head, as excitement bubbles. "Yes, dear. I will do whatever you want me to do."

"You can't die on me, babe. You can't die on Blake," he quivers as tears form in his eyes.

I take a seat on his lap and wrap my arms around him. "I'm not going anywhere. I know it will be ok, and that this is the right thing. You have to put your trust in me, and in my body. Everything will be just fine."

Trying but Not Trying

On October 5th I get my period, right on schedule. My dad is having a major surgery at the end of the month, so we have decided to put a hold on getting pregnant until next year. I know in my heart that if anything happens to him, and he doesn't make it through, I might miscarry the baby from stress alone.

Almost two weeks later, after a severe ice storm, I walk outside to dump leftovers on the compost pile, when I slip on the algae covered wood that lines the flowerbed.

Knives shoot through my back and down my legs. Intense pain overtakes my entire pelvis like a burning fire. Lying on my back in the mulch, I roll onto my stomach and attempt to push up to a stance. Unable to force myself through the pain, my arms give out and I drop face first into the wet mulch.

"Please!" I yell. "Shawn, help!"

Shawn hears my screams from inside the house and, within seconds, he bullets out of the door and rushes to my side. Scooping me gently in his arms, he carries my wet and ragged body inside.

"Something is broken!" I scream through tears. "I can't move!"

I can tell by the look on his face, that he's terrified. His eyes are wider than I've ever seen. The blue irises are cloudy from tears, and his mouth hangs open.

"What can I do, babe? Do you need to go to the hospital?" he asks.

Blake appears from behind him, tears streaming down her face. I notice her fear, and I take a deep breath to try and calm myself. 'Mom mode' takes over— I need to be stronger than this— I need her to know it's going to be ok.

Three deep breaths and I'm able to speak. "Get me a pillow and an ice pack. I'm not throwing up, so maybe I didn't break it. Everyone always says you throw up when you break something." I don't remember who told me that, but in this moment, it's keeping me from panicking. Maybe it isn't even true, but right now it's enough.

The throbbing continues, and the pressure from the ice pack is unbearable against my tailbone. Once I begin to settle, and the adrenaline fades, I notice the intense swelling in my right knee as well.

"My damn knee, too," I say to Shawn. "Stupid thing dislocated in the fall. I'll need to ice it."

Shawn runs to the kitchen for another ice pack as my tears turn to anger. My body is such a failure. Just as I was beginning to trust it again, it completely gives out on me. I bite my lip to keep from saying words Blake shouldn't hear, and grip the cushion of the couch, squeezing it tightly every time I move.

Blake's tiny body hesitantly takes a seat next to me. "Mommy, are you ok?" she asks.

My heart aches for her. I hate that she has to see me this way. Your parents are supposed to be invincible, and I know how hard it is when you realize they aren't.

I swallow my pain, and pull her in. "Mommy will be ok, sweetie. Don't you worry."

I readjust my butt on a pillow and try to get comfortable. Shawn brings me a glass of water and two pain-killers. I hate drugs, and refuse to take it most of the time, but this is a necessity.

[92]

I feel the pills slide down my throat and anxiety builds as they hit my stomach. I've never been good with medication.

"What if I react? Will they make me loopy? I need to take care of Blake, I can't be drugged up," I whine to Shawn.

"They are low dose, babe. They won't knock you out. Even if they did, I called out of work— I'll take care of Blake. You need to rest and see how you feel in the morning."

I turn on the television to cartoons and curl up with Blake under a blanket. The throbbing in my back starts to dissipate, and I drift off to sleep.

✳✳✳✳✳

Whenever I ovulate, I am blessed with the pain of middlesmertz. I'm aware, down to the minute, when the egg is being pushed out of the ovary. This has worked well for us in learning the process of NFP. Unfortunately, with my recent fall, middlesmertz is nearly unrecognizable. This is the first cycle that I am forced to guess when my fertile window is.

I hobble around for four days until I finally start to feel like myself again. My knee has started to bear weight and the swelling has diminished. Although it still painful to sit on my tailbone, I can function pretty well. Luckily, I didn't have to worry about abstaining from sex during ovulation—my injury did that for me.

A few nights pass, and Shawn and I decide to do the deed. Since it is post-ovulation, the condoms are left in the nightstand. I'm on day 19 of my cycle, and should be about four or five days passed ovulation. During the encounter, I immediately regret my decision as the pain once again radiates throughout my pelvis. Knives shoot through my entire bottom, and I rush Shawn to finish before it gets too painful to handle.

"Sorry babe, I just can't," I cry.

"Why didn't you tell me to stop," he scolds. "I feel awful. I'm so sorry."

I hover in pain on all fours while he fetches an ice pack from the freezer. I realize it was too early to try and have sex, and will be regretting the decision for days to come.

✳✳✳✳✳

Two weeks pass, and we are on our way to visit my dad in the hospital while he is recovering from the surgery. He had complications the doctors had trouble controlling, and for a while, I didn't think he would make it through. I'm thankful we decided to put off trying for a baby, a baby I could potentially lose if the stress of my father's death took over.

Mom is driving and Blake is in the back napping in her car seat. An overwhelming sense of nausea hits me out of nowhere.

"Do you have a bag?" I ask. "Or, maybe I need you to pull over."

Mom looks at me. "Car sick?"

I nod my head.

She rips the bag off the shifter and hands it to me. "Try and chew some gum, or open the window. That usually helps."

I do as she says and the nausea slowly subsides. I've gotten car sick my whole life, so this is nothing new. I'm not sure if it's the stress from Dad's recovery, the heat, or the traffic, but I need to get out of this car.

Once we arrive at the hospital, my stomach is still uneasy. Standing in the parking lot, I stare at the windows of the building and imagine the thousands of sick and dying people behind them. Somewhere, someone could be taking their last breath. A man could be told he's only got six weeks to live; a mother being informed that her baby has passed.

And with the onset of a panic attack, the nausea hits again.

I take Blake's hand and follow Mom inside. The elevator music doesn't help ease my mind, and deep breaths are all that's keeping the vomit in my stomach. We arrive at the ICU, and a wave of anxiety hits me before we enter. I prepare myself for how he will look and how I will feel seeing him in that condition.

What if Blake asks questions or feels uncomfortable? What if I can't hold it together and it scares her?

I take one more deep breath, slide a new piece of gum in my mouth, and enter the room.

[94]

My father sits in the chair. His color is grey and his glasses hang by a thread on the end of his nose as he glances up at me. His soft blue eyes stick out like a sore thumb against his white hair and beige gown.

"Hello there, daughter," he says in a soft, but chipper voice.

"Hi, Pappy," Blake chirps as she hesitantly moves in for a hug.

I can't control it— tears stream down my face at the sight of him. He's so frail and weak— very different from the father I've grown to love; Mr. invincible.

"How are you feeling?" I struggle to get out, fighting with my emotions.

"Oh, I'm hanging in there. Ready to get out of here," he chuckles.

I'm pleasantly surprised by his mood.

"I bet," I respond, wiping the two tears away that snuck down my cheek before he notices.

As mom monopolizes the conversation, I lie down on the couch by the window. My stomach still isn't right, and the wavering nausea has decided to return.

"Maybe you're hungry," Mom adds.

I haven't eaten today and food sounds strangely tempting. I ask dad if he wants anything, and then Blake and I head to the cafeteria for lunch. A half-hour later we return with a colossal amount of food.

"Hungry?" Dad asks with a deep laugh.

I smile, "Seems so."

Thankfully, eating sends my nausea packing. Maybe it is the stress on an empty stomach that's making me sick, and now that I've seen Dad, I feel a little better. The doctor explains that he may be here a while yet, but has hope that everything will work out just fine. We visit for a few hours before heading home. Luckily, the nausea dissipates for the rest of the day, and I don't think about it again.

"Your father has to go to Philadelphia to get a procedure done to deal with complications from the surgery. He's supposed to leave tomorrow evening. The ambulance will take him."

I listen to her explain, while I count the days on the calendar. November 5th.

Tomorrow is November 5th?

I flip the page back to October to validate my last period—October 5th.

"I'm late," I blurt out.

"What?" Mom asks. "Late for what?"

"Nothing," I respond. "I gotta go. I'll talk to you later."

As I count the days on the calendar again, I realize that I'm several days passed my period. I hadn't even noticed because of everything going on with Dad.

Maybe it was stress? Maybe it was the fall that threw my cycle off?

As I run everything through my head, my phone rings. I answer it before I check the caller ID.

"We are pregnant!" My sister-in-law yells through the speaker.

"Wait, what? Who is pregnant?" I ask, confused.

"Me, silly!" she responds.

"Oh my God! Congratulations!" I yell. She and my brother have been trying to get pregnant for quite a while, and although the timing isn't great, I'm so happy for them. Maybe this will give Dad something to push for—something to give him the will to hang on a little longer.

We talk for a while. After hanging up, I dig through the baskets under the sink to see if I have any leftover pregnancy tests hiding in the back—nothing.

I throw a coat on Blake and we escape to the dollar store. Three tests and two candy bars slide down the conveyor belt as I impatiently tap my finger on the metal.

"Anything else?" the cashier asks, silently judging me.

I want to say something snotty, but I remain professional.

"That's all for today, thanks."

Ripping open the candy bar and shoving it in my mouth on the way out, I snarl at her.

She's afraid of this hormone driven mother, I can tell.

I hurry home, anxious to take the test but I don't have to pee.

Great, now I have to wait.

Any woman will tell you that waiting sucks. Waiting the two weeks to ovulate sucks— waiting the two weeks to test sucks— waiting the two minutes for the stick to change colors sucks— and waiting nine months for a baby to be born sucks. But, get used to it, motherhood is all about waiting.

After tucking Blake into bed, I decide to wait until morning to test. I want to be confident in the results—no questions—and I know first morning urine is the most concentrated.

Millions of thoughts fly through my mind as I toss and turn for hours.

What if I am pregnant? What if something happens to Dad? What if I miscarry because of the stress? What if I get Preeclampsia again? What if I die?

Finally, I pass out.

✳✳✳✳✳

Blake awakens me in the morning by climbing on my stomach to give me hugs, accentuating my urge to pee. I remember about the test and leap out of bed.

"What's wrong, Mommy?" she asks.

"Nothing, sweetie. Mommy just really has to pee."

After flipping the television on, and handing Blake a granola bar, I hide in the bathroom for a little while.

The dollar store tests aren't the fancy kind that you pee on. Instead, you need to use a dropper and transfer your urine from a cup, onto the stick. I have never mastered this, and usually end up with pee all over my bathroom counter. Today is no exception. You

[97]

need to—1. Pee in a cup. 2. Put pee cup on counter. 3. Dip syringe in pee to suck it up. 4. Squirt pee on the little hole at the end of the test. 5. Wait for results while wiping up pee you dropped everywhere.

The only common denominator between all the different types of tests? The waiting. Some women prefer to hide the test, or cover the label. I, on the other hand, prefer to stare directly at it without blinking. It's like an adrenaline rush, watching the paper turn dark as my urine glides across it.

Within seconds, I watch the control line go dark. A few moments later, it's there—clear as day—a second line. There are no doubts here, no questioning whether it's an evaporation line, or a faulty test—it is positive.

I sit down on the toilet and take a deep breath. I'm not shaking like I did the first time. My chest doesn't tighten and I'm not breaking out in a cold sweat. I am calm, relaxed, and actually a little excited!

I hear the back door close and wrap the test in toilet paper, carrying it out to the kitchen where Shawn has just gotten home from work.

"Here," I say, handing the wad of paper to him.

"Ew," he says. "What is that?"

"Just look at it," I respond.

He unwraps the paper and his eyes widen. "How? When? You're pregnant?" he questions.

"Yeah, I guess I ovulated late. It looks like you're going to be a daddy again!"

A smile illuminates his face and he wraps his arms around me. I breathe in the happiness, allowing no room for fear.

This is going to be wonderful.

Dad is due for surgery the following day—a surgery that will save his life if it's successful. I know it is early to share the news, and I would prefer to wait the entire 12 weeks, but this is an exception.

I dial the number to the hospital and sit in Blake's room, staring out the window at the snow flurries that have begun to fall.

"Hello?" his tired voice answers.

"Hi, Dad," I respond.

"Well, hello daughter. I wasn't expecting a call from you."

"I know," I start. "I just wanted to share some good news with you."

"Oh," he cuts me off. "Your brother already called me. They are having a baby. It's so exciting."

"Yes, yes it is. But, that isn't what I wanted to tell you," I explain.

"Is everything ok?" he asks, his tone quickly shifting.

I nod my head as if he can see me, "Everything is wonderful," I respond. "I'm pregnant."

The phone is silent, until I hear his voice crack on the other end. "That is wonderful," he says through muffled tears. "Really, really wonderful."

Drops of joy fall down my cheeks, too. If this is the last time I talk to him, at least I know that he knew. I can hear the nurse in the background preparing him for the big day, and I say my goodbyes, hoping it's only temporary.

"Love you, Dad."

"I love you too, daughter. And, congratulations! I'm so happy to be a grandpa again."

✳✳✳✳✳

My father's surgery is successful and he finally gets to come home from the hospital a week later. I am combating unbearable morning sickness, and every hour of the day is spent tirelessly avoiding throwing up.

Luckily, I never actually allow myself to vomit. On a list of things I hate most in this world— throwing up is pretty high, and I avoid it at all costs. It's one of those things that I truly believe is mind over matter. I refuse to allow it to happen, so it doesn't.

Homeschooling Blake has become exhausting. Brushing my hair is draining. Cooking dinner is the equivalent of running a marathon. I am dog-tired five minutes after I wake up. I hate to admit it, but I'm starting to resent this tiny human growing inside of me, and I just want to feel normal again.

At around six weeks, I struggle to relax in a bath. An hour prior, I was wishing I had never gotten pregnant because of how awful I felt. Now, I am dealing with the guilt of it. I sit and stare at my stomach, making conversation with the tiny embryo. I know the placenta is still forming, and that it's the major influence in Preeclampsia. I place my hands on my belly, forming a heart with my fingers.

"You will build an amazing placenta little baby. You will grow strong and healthy. Mommy will make you a nice home. I'm sorry I was mad at you for making me feel sick, I didn't mean it."

If talking to plants has been scientifically proven to help them grow, why can't talking to my baby?

Doctor Do—Doctor Don't

Now that I am seven weeks pregnant, I know I need to find a different doctor and schedule an appointment. Standing outside of the viewing window at Blake's dance class, I eavesdrop on some other mom's birthing experiences.

"I had a homebirth with my second, and it was incredible. I would never birth in a hospital again." she explains, her eyes lighting up.

Another mom questions, "Does the doctor come to you?"

"It's a midwife, and she only delivers at homes—not in the hospital. She's been doing it for many years, and is trained to handle almost all emergency situations. She was great."

I stealthily inch closer, hoping to stay unnoticed.

"Women forget that birth is natural. We are given everything we need, we just overlook that. Women are afraid—we don't trust our bodies."

I'm intrigued by her story, and her points are making a lot of sense. One of the other moms walks away, seemingly offended or annoyed by the conversation.

I chime in, "Can you tell me more about this?" I ask. "I had a horrendous first delivery, and we are looking at options if we have another in the future. I never thought about a home birth."

[101]

"Sure," she responds. "I can tell you whatever you want to know!"

My ears perk, chewing every word she spits out.

"Here's my midwife's name and number," the other mom says as she writes it down on the back of a business card. "Call her, tell her Lena sent you. She can answer any questions you have when you guys are ready to start trying."

I thank her for the information as the kids exit class and Blake monopolizes my attention. I really like her, and everything she believes in, and hope we can chat more in the future.

Upon arriving home, I run the info by Shawn.

"So, how about a home birth?" I ask

His face turns to displeasure and disgust.

"What if something happens?" he asks, shaking his head. "We aren't in a hospital. What if it's like last time? You would've died if we would've been at home. You and Blake. There's no way this is even an option for us."

He makes good arguments. Home birth is very scary to me. In fact, birth in general is terrifying. Once you have a traumatic experience, it's hard to look at things any other way. Women who go through something like I did, never get over it. It leaves an imprint in your mind similar to PTSD. The "what if's" control your thoughts, and you thank your lucky stars that the doctors saved your life.

But, did they?

I need to do more research. For hours, I look into birthing options. Home births vs. birthing centers and hospitals. Doctors vs. midwives. Medicated vs. un-medicated. Vaginal vs. cesarean.

I want to be informed this time. If there's one thing I learned, it's that I'm not allowing someone else to make these decisions for me ever again. I am going to be an advocate for myself during this pregnancy, but I need to be educated.

Women forget that we are in charge of our pregnancies and deliveries. **Ultimately, every decision is ours and ours alone.** Doctors can advise us, midwives can guide us, our spouses can support us—but this is OUR choice.

[102]

So, what do I want?

I want a home birth, in my bathroom tub. I want roses floating on the surface of the water and drops of Lavender circulating through the air from my diffuser. I want Shawn rubbing my shoulders and applying a cool rag to my forehead. I want to eat and drink during labor and walk barefoot in the grass outside. I want Blake to be as much of a part of it as she would like, or be able to run around outside if she gets bored.

Using the phone number I got from Lena, I call the midwife. After some brief chatting, I inquire about her availability in July.

"I have one other delivery booked so far, but as long as you pay now, I can hold your spot. My fee is three-thousand."

I swallow down a breath. "Three thousand?" I repeat back to her.

Our insurance deductible is two-thousand, so what's another grand on top of it?

"Now," she starts. "Tell me about your first pregnancy. All normal, right? Vaginal or cesarean delivery?"

"Well, actually I had Preeclampsia and was induced at 36 weeks. Vaginally delivered."

"No, no," she responds. "I can't do your homebirth because you're high risk. I'm sorry. I can recommend an OBGYN if you would like?"

Questions run through my mind, but I don't ask any of them. "Um, ok? Go ahead."

I write down the name and number and say goodbye. Taking a seat on the bed with a sweaty piece of paper in my hand, disappointment floods my mind.

When Shawn arrives home from work, I fill him in.

"I feel better with you delivering in the hospital," he admits. "Especially with everything that happened last time. I just don't feel comfortable with a home birth, I'm sorry."

I agree. Until I heard the words "high risk" out loud, I didn't feel the fear. I imagined a beautiful—complication free— delivery, but what if it wasn't? What if I had to be transferred and paid the 3k,

[103]

and the 2k deductible, too? Money is always a big deciding factor in our life decisions. And I felt ignorant for not looking at these facts sooner.

After realizing it is for the best, and a home birth never should've been on the table for us, I call the number of the OBGYN she gave me and set up an appointment.

The First Appointment Jitters

At nine weeks along, I have my first appointment with the OB that Lena's midwife referred. The building is quaint. It is an old Victorian house that has been renovated into a doctor's office.

Small flowers float on the wallpaper around the room and the heater vent kicks out warm air against my ankles. I begin reading a pamphlet sitting next to me as the secretary calls my name to fill out paperwork.

"This is your first appointment, right?" she asks.

I nod my head.

"I'll need your insurance cards to make copies."

I dig them out of my wallet and hand them to her before taking a seat next to Shawn.

"I'm nervous," I whisper.

He grabs my hand with his. "It'll be ok, babe. Deep breath."

Before I can finish the sheet, a brown-haired lady calls my name without looking up from her paper. Tiny, black-framed glasses rest on the edge of her nose.

"Come on back," she directs. Looking up, she drops the glasses off her face and allows them to dangle on her neck from the end of a tether.

[105]

We follow her to the first room on the right.

"Ok, let's get a weight on you."

I step on the scale. The number is ten pounds less than I weighed prior to getting pregnant.

"Morning sickness has really taken it out of me this time around," I explain. "Most days I feel like I ran a marathon. Zero appetite. Zero ambition."

Her expressionless face stares back at me. I become uneasy and start rambling.

"Is that normal? To feel sick like this? I mean, I had Preeclampsia with my first and I know ..."

"It's normal," she cuts me off. "Make sure you're taking your vitamins and try to eat. Sometimes eating makes you less nauseous. Any questions?"

I shake my head.

Everything feels so rushed. I have questions—hundreds of questions. But, she is making me feel unwelcomed.

Is she busy? Is that why she's pushing me out the door? There wasn't anyone else in the waiting room, though. Maybe her shift is ending? I better not take up too much more of her time.

"No, I guess not."

I hate this feeling. I want things to be different this time and I'm obviously at the wrong office for that to happen.

"The doctor will do an ultrasound in two weeks to get an idea of a due date. He will make sure there is a heartbeat and everything," she says as she practically pushes us out the door. "Sharon can schedule that for you."

I stand at the desk, baffled. Thousands of questions stream through my mind as I try to digest what just happened. Shawn senses my stress and schedules the appointment for me.

"Ok, we will see you guys in two weeks. Take care."

The door shuts and the crisp air floats through my hair. I tighten my jacket around my bloated belly and scurry to the car.

[106]

Once inside, I let it out. "What the hell? Could she have sucked anymore?!" I yell. "She was a bitch! She didn't give two shits about me, or my baby, or my past! Why would anyone hire someone like that?"

Shawn stares at me.

"What? Why aren't you saying anything?"

"I don't know what to say. What do you want to do? Find another doctor?"

I sit in silence.

"Maybe it's just her— maybe the doctor is better. Why not give him a chance? If you still aren't happy, we will look for someone else," Shawn finishes.

I feel defeated. Shawn puts the car in gear and drives off. I know I have a while yet before I really need a doctor, but I want it now. I want to begin forming this imaginary relationship where everything is rainbows and butterflies. Where he knows me by my name when I walk in, and I don't need to explain my traumatic history at every single appointment.

I stare out the window as Blake sings lullabies in the background.

Shawn reaches over and wraps my hand in his. "Let's just see what happens in two weeks."

✶✶✶✶✶

"Ryan?" A young woman calls from the doorway. I'm thankful for her blonde hair bouncing on the tops of her shoulders. A sense of calm takes over once I realize it's a different nurse than last time. I let a loud sigh of relief slip out between my lips.

"Yes." I stand up. Pulling my shirt over my—not yet baby—belly, I follow her to the back room.

"Ok, my name is Daria—I'm Dr. Paul's nurse. I will see you on some of your appointments. I'm going to go over the basic stuff with you, and then the doctor will come in and do the ultrasound. Is that ok?"

I nod my head. "Yes, that sounds good."

[107]

"Why don't you step on the scale here? We will get a weight on you."

The number hasn't changed. I still don't have much of an appetite, and literally have to force myself to eat throughout the day.

The only things I manage to keep down are the sixteen different kinds of prenatal vitamins I've tried—all of which bother me in some way. After reacting to six of them, I decide to eat a balanced diet instead and hope it will be enough. When the nurse asks, I simply nod my head and agree.

Yes, I take my prenatal like a good girl.

"Have a seat. How have you been feeling? If you have morning sickness it should start to calm down pretty soon. Let's talk about your health history. It says you had Preeclampsia?"

I nod my head, "Yeah, I was induced at 36 weeks."

"That must've been very scary for you," she states, sympathetically. "Can you tell me more about it?"

Surprised by her intrigue, I explain the details of my delivery. Tears begin to coat my eyes while I talk. I refuse to blink, allowing any of them to escape onto my cheek.

Sensing my distress, she slides her chair over to the edge of the bed and places her hand on my thigh. "It'll be ok. Please, don't be afraid. Dr. Paul is amazing. He will take excellent care of you and your baby."

I love you already.

"Can you deliver my baby?" I ask, before my brain has a chance to filter the words.

She laughs, "I wish. I don't deliver. I don't have my license for that. I can do everything else, though."

She asks me a few more questions before checking my vitals and leaving the room.

"She was nice," Shawn states, awaiting my conclusion.

"She was very sweet," I agree.

The door opens and a hand pushes toward me.

"You must be Ryan? I'm Dr. Paul. It's very nice to meet you."

My sweaty palm matches his and we exchange a shake. I glance into brown eyes, scanning his face quickly, being sure not to hold the gaze too long.

"Nice to meet you. This is my husband, Shawn."

"Hello, Shawn. I'm Dr. Paul. Don't worry; I'm going to take good care of your wife and baby."

Shawn lends a wink in my direction as Dr. Paul takes a seat on the rolling stool and reads over my paperwork.

"Preeclampsia, huh?"

I nod.

"Don't worry. Most often it's a first pregnancy phenomenon. We will watch for it, but you should be ok. Take a deep breath; you're doing great so far. Now, should we take a look at your baby?"

I lie back and lift my shirt up, exposing my still-flat stomach. He squirts a cold blue gel onto it, and then presses the wand down. His machine is old, and the screen quality is poor—at best. Very different from what I was used to seeing in my first pregnancy.

"Ok. So, here is your baby," he points to the screen.

A very apparent picture of a tiny embryo fills the blurred background —*Two arms, two legs, and a big head.* .

A smile extends from ear to ear. "And, the placenta?" I blurt out.

Dr. Paul breaks his gaze from the screen and places his free hand on top of mine.

"Ryan, listen to me. Everything will be fine. Your baby looks great and is measuring right where it should. You're on your way to a very beautiful—complication free—pregnancy."

I can feel my heart rate drop and my breathing slow as the anxiety begins to flee.

"I'm going to send you for your 12-week bloodwork. Did you have this in your first pregnancy? It is optional, but it'll show us if you have any markers for the Preeclampsia. The Perinatologist will perform that, along with a scan. Pairing the results will give you enough information to see what your risks are."

"Write me a script," I agree, knowing how desperately I crave the results.

He hands us a picture of our little peanut, and we head to the car. Blake insists on holding it while I secure the seatbelt over her shoulder.

Shawn stares at me from the driver's seat. "So?" he inquires.

"I love him!" I squeal!

Genetic Testing—Again

Weeks drag along when you're pregnant. You're constantly looking toward the next big thing. The next appointment. The next ultrasound. The next exam. Anything and everything revolves around this tiny human growing inside of you. You are at their mercy, and don't trust anyone who tries to convince you otherwise.

At twelve weeks, we sit in the waiting room of Dr. Paul's colleague, Dr. Volgo, a Perinatologist at one of the local hospitals. Nerves soar through my body as I remember the last time we did this, and all of the emotions I had when we were told about the possibility of Down syndrome. Soon enough, I will know if Preeclampsia is going to rear its ugly head again. I begin to question my decision to find out and wonder if perhaps ignorance really is bliss.

A nurse with a pixie haircut calls me back before I can retreat. I take a seat in a recliner, and she rubs an alcohol wipe over my inner elbow. Tying a rubber band around my bicep, she instructs me to make a fist while she readies the needle.

My nerves are shot in my arms from all the tubes of blood taken in the hospital five years ago, so I don't even flinch when the cold metal pierces my skin. The vials fill, but I stare out the window instead of watching the blood pool in the tiny glass canisters.

"Ok, we are all set. Hold pressure on it there. Takes a few weeks for this type of test, did your doctor tell you that?"

"Yeah," I respond while holding the gauze with two fingers.

She applies tape to the wound and I pull my sleeve down.

"You can follow me to the ultrasound room. The tech is waiting."

Once in the room, the tech squeezes that familiar blue gel on my stomach.

It's warmed here, as opposed to the freezing ice at Dr. Paul's. I stare at the screen, awaiting our tiny baby's appearance. At last, the screen clears and a grey head is visible.

"Did the doctor explain what we are looking for?"

"Yes," I respond. "Well, kinda. I've been through this before. They told us our first daughter had Down syndrome, but recanted after the ultrasound."

The tech raises her eyebrows and seems unsure of how to respond.

"Dr. Paul said we will be able to tell my likelihood for a recurring Preeclampsia by these tests—otherwise we wouldn't have done them."

My talking has elicited no response from her as she silently continues to move the wand around my belly and push buttons on the machine.

I look at Shawn, who is staring at her. His eyes burn through the stale air. "Is that correct?" he questions, in a tone I've never heard from him prior.

She halts, and turns toward us, finally acknowledging our existence.

"Yes. But, you seem to have already known all of this."

Condescending bitch.

I want to say so much, but I bite my tongue when Shawn's hand presses down on my shin.

[112]

"And, last time the doctors tried to convince us that our daughter had Down syndrome before they were sure. So, you can understand our questioning," he explains.

His attitude is a major turn on. If I wasn't pregnant already, it would be soon to occur.

"I understand," she responds, defensively. "It must be a very stressful time for you both. I will do my best to explain things."

"Thank you," I mutter, matching her tone.

For the next 30 minutes, she examines certain markers on the baby and placenta. Once completed, she hands me a few pictures and covers my stomach with a towel.

"The doctor will be in shortly to go over the results."

After she exits, Shawn and I whisper about how rude she was as we stare at the pictures of our baby. Only a few minutes pass before the door opens again and a small bald man walks through.

"Hello Ryan, I'm Dr. Volgo. Let's discuss your results and then go over any questions you may have. Does that sound ok?"

I nod my head while he shakes Shawn's hand, introducing himself again.

"Dr. Paul has let me know about your history of Preeclampsia, and the tech filled me in about your previous genetic testing in your first pregnancy. Now, let's go over the results from your testing here."

He holds a paper in front of me and begins explaining.

"Now, the blood test will show if you have certain markers for Preeclampsia. As you know, similar markers can show for both Pre-e and Downs, hence the reason the doctors assumed your first child had it."

I had read about that in my research, but it was nice to hear confirmation on it from a real doctor. Validation always makes my anxiety diminish.

"Well, you could possibly have some markers for Preeclampsia, which means there's a possibility you could end up with it again. We won't know until we get the bloodwork."

[113]

My heart sinks and my stomach drops while I break out in a cold sweat. Shawn shifts from the chair to his feet and joins me at my side, holding my hand.

"But, your ultrasound is perfect. Your placenta looks beautiful and I would say your risk of recurrence is low. Maybe 10-15%. I'm going to recommend starting you on a blood thinner. Do you know about this?"

"Yes, they had me on it with my first," I respond as I wipe my sweaty hands on my jeans, breaking the hold with Shawn.

"One baby –dose of blood thinner a day until about 35 weeks. It'll help with blood flow."

I nod my head, "Ok."

He explains a few more things, but I zone out and think about the 10-15% chance of getting Preeclampsia. It means I have 85-90% chance of not getting it at all! Joy illuminates my body and I float on air as I follow Shawn out of the office.

On the way home, we stop at the pharmacy to purchase the pills. I read the bottle before popping one in my mouth.

PREGNANT OR BREASTFEEDING WOMEN SHOULD CONSULT A PHYSICIAN BEFORE USE.

Something about this bothers me, but I don't think Dr. Volgo would've recommended it if it was in any way harmful. However, my gut convinces me to do a little research before introducing it to my system.

Even though I find cons to taking it, the fear of Preeclampsia negates them all. I swallow the tiny pill and then slide the ultrasound pictures into a photo album sitting on the dresser that stands alone in the nursery.

✳✳✳✳✳

"Do you see this?" I ask Shawn as I lift my shirt and point to my stomach.

"Yes," he responds. "What is it?"

"I think it's a rash," I explain, concerned. "Maybe from the blood thinner? It's the only thing new."

He shakes his head. "I guess your gut was right, again. You gonna keep taking it?"

Now, I'm trapped by indecision. "I'll call the doctor and see what he thinks."

After explaining my situation to the nurse on the other end, she tells me to stop the medication. A rash is a signal of an allergic reaction and not something to take lightly. I hesitantly agree, and toss it in the trash. A slight sense of relief escalates through my body, but is quickly followed by nerves.

Now, there is nothing to keep the Preeclampsia at bay. My blood pressure will definitely elevate without it.

"I didn't like you taking it anyway," Shawn yells from the living room. "I read it can cause miscarriage in early pregnancy—not sure if it's true, but it's not something I want to find out."

His research impresses me and I gloat a little as I walk through the living room. "Trying to be like me, huh?"

"I also read that eating spicy food can help blood flow, so why don't we try that instead?" he adds.

I take a seat next to him on the couch and Blake slides in between us. As a tiny family of three, we enjoy an afternoon of cuddling as the snowflakes coat the ground outside.

It's A...

At 20 weeks, we are back at Dr. Volgo's for our anatomy scan and detailed bloodwork results. The nurse had called me a few weeks ago, but didn't explain much—just that there were some things Dr. Volgo wanted to discuss at our next appointment.

As the door opens, Shawn and I count our blessings when a red-haired tech walks through the door; we aren't stuck with the condescending snob from our last visit.

She bounces over to the chair and immediately engages us in conversation. "I'm Lori. I'm going to be doing your scan today. You look so cute with your little belly," she says as she taps my stomach. "I'm going to take a lot of measurements to check for any abnormalities or deformities. I see your daughter there," she says, pointing to Blake, "so you guys know what this is about. Now, do you want to know the gender?"

"Yes," I blurt out. I've never had patience, and it's been driving me insane not knowing for this long already. "We are pretty convinced it's a boy," I add, trying to pass the time as she begins the scan with measurements of the baby's skull.

"Any particular reason?" she inquires.

"Not really. Just, that this pregnancy is so different from my first. A lot of morning sickness, and fatigue—just, a lot different."

I shift glances from the screen to my belly as I feel the butterfly movements inside. A week ago, I finally began to look pregnant. A tiny baby bump had appeared practically overnight, and I was excited to slide into the maternity pants I had bought at the thrift shop.

"Do you feel your baby move?" she asks.

"Yeah. I have been for quite a while. Way earlier this time. Probably around 12-14 weeks was the first time I felt the tiny flutters. Everyone kept telling me it was just gas, but I disagree."

She laughs, "It's very hard to tell sometimes."

"Here are the four chambers of the heart. What a great heart. Very healthy. I'm excited to show the doctor, it's not often we get such a beautiful functioning heart like this. Wow!"

I'm taken aback.

Is it really that great? Why is it so great? Are normal hearts sub-par? Was Blake's heart bad? Why didn't I ever ask about it?

"Is that good?" I can hear the insecurity in my voice. "I mean, you seem surprised that it's so good. Like, is it too good?"

She laughs, again, "It's perfect. No need to worry. Everything looks beautiful so far."

So far.

I know we have the placenta left. It is fully formed now, and if it shows any abnormalities it will mean that Preeclampsia is definitely in the future.

"You guys ready for the gender?"

I shut my mind off and concentrate on the screen.

"This is a great shot. Do you guys kno--"

"It's a girl!" I cut her off.

"Yes! Congrats you guys. It seems your guess was wrong," she giggles. "You had a 50/50 shot."

Shawn looks disappointed. He was so hyped up to have a boy, and we were convinced that it was. We knew my sister-in-law was having a girl because of the 12 week blood work, and something in us wanted to be different.

[118]

I sympathetically stare into his eyes. Once he notices, he reaches out and holds my hand. "Another beautiful little girl ... I guess we will have to figure out a name," he smiles.

I clutch his hand as the love in my heart grows stronger— this man amazes me every single day.

Snapping us back to reality, the nurse interrupts our moment.

"Ok, so the placenta looks good but its location is troublesome. Currently, it's covering your cervix. If it stays there, you'll need a cesarean."

"A cesarean?" I question.

"Yes. You can't deliver vaginally with placenta previa. There are just too many risks. The doctor will go over all of this with you. Other than that your scan looks very good. I'm going to send him in. He may want to take a look."

Once again, I'm worried. Worry should be my middle name at this point because pregnancy is exhausting. The women that have uncomplicated pregnancies have no idea how lucky they are. There are literally thousands of issues that can occur at any time in your 40 weeks, and it's absolutely terrifying.

The doctor enters a few moments later. He shakes our hands and takes a seat.

"I'm just going to take a quick look," he explains as he squeezes more gel onto my stomach. "Ok, yes. The placenta is low. We will have to watch it. A lot of times they move on their own as the pregnancy progresses. Nothing to worry about yet."

I'm slightly relieved, but once I get a thought in my mind, it never really goes away. I like to be prepared for catastrophic situations. My therapist always said it was a symptom of my anxiety. You picture the worst case scenario so that you can prepare your mind, that way you believe nothing can really be that bad. I start picturing a C-section and how much I do not want one.

"Ok, thank you," Shawn responds when he notices my mind wandering.

"Yes, thank you," I mimic.

After asking some questions and scheduling our next appointment, we leave the office with a handful of pictures of our little girl. On the ride home we begin tossing name ideas at each other, unable to agree on one just yet.

Gestational Diabetes is no Joke

Visiting Dr. Paul has become a monthly thing over the course of my pregnancy. By the third visit, I question why he has never tested my urine.

"Can't trust it," he explains. "Hydration can skew those results so dramatically. I do want to schedule a 24 hour on you though, just to get your baseline. Do you have a jug?"

"Not anymore," I respond. "I know how to do it though."

He opens the cabinet and pulls an orange jug from it. From a separate spot, he retrieves a white plastic hat to catch the urine.

"Do it this week and drop it off. I'll have the results at your next appointment then."

I grab the stuff and hand it to Shawn.

"Blood pressure looks great and your weight is perfect. How have you been feeling?" Dr. Paul asks while squeezing my ankles to check for swelling.

"Well, I do have one problem," I start. "When my arms hang, my veins get huge. Like the size of a pencil. Is this normal?"

"I'm not sure. Can you show me?" he inquires.

I stand and allow my arms to hang at my sides. Almost instantly, my veins pool with blood and expand to five times their normal size.

"It's almost like varicose," he says. "I think it's just because there's so much more blood volume in pregnant women, and because your veins are already close to the surface. Yes, they become much more pronounced. Do you have any pain?" he asks.

I shake my head. "I wouldn't say pain, it's just uncomfortable feeling. Tight like."

As I explain, he lifts my hand above my head and the veins return to normal.

"That's a good sign. Yeah, let's just keep an eye on it. But, I think it's ok. Just another annoying pregnancy thing."

I take a seat on the table and lie back, lifting my shirt and rolling down the band on my pants. Dr. Paul has a student with him today and allows her to attempt locating my baby's heartbeat.

Minutes pass and panic slowly fills the young girl's face. I feed on her emotion and can feel the anxiety building throughout my body.

"Is everything ok?" I beg. "Can't you find it? It's got to be there."

Dr. Paul rips the monitor from her hand and presses it onto my belly. With the other hand, he pushes around trying to determine how the baby is positioned. Within seconds, a rhythmic beat is heard.

"144 beats per minutes. Good strong heart," he encourages. "Take a deep breath, Ryan. Everything is ok."

I shift from fear to anger. "Maybe you should learn how to use that thing. You're gonna give someone a heart attack," I scold her.

Overrun with fear and guilt, she cowers in the corner and I immediately regret my outburst.

"I'm sorry, I didn't mean to yell. I just already have enough stress on this pregnancy."

She apologizes profusely, "I'm so sorry. So, so, sorry. It's my first day here. I've only used it a few times. Please, I'm sorry."

Dr. Paul rubs my arm to calm me down as Shawn massages my feet.

"Well, she probably won't be back," he whispers in my ear.

Anger turns to nervous laughter, and I allow her to try again. Dr. Paul demonstrates how to palpate my stomach and find the position of the baby before engaging the machine. Once she does, the heartbeat is heard almost immediately.

"There it is," she exclaims. "I'm so sorry about before. I didn't mean to scare you like that."

I smile, but I'm still aggravated at her ignorance. After having Blake, I know I don't want any students in my delivery room, but I didn't realize they would be at my regular appointments too.

I pull Dr. Paul aside and brief him on my wishes. He agrees, and makes no hesitation in jotting it down on my paperwork.

"Now we need to do the diabetes test. You did this with your first, I'm sure," he explains while handing me a script. "Between 24-26 weeks, ok?"

I remember the drink well. It tasted like drinking an orange soda that sat out for four hours and went flat, and then someone dumped 15 packets of sugar into it. It was disgusting, and I was sure I didn't want to put it in mine, or my baby's, body.

"Do I have any other option besides the drink?" I ask. "I'm allergic to some food dyes and I know it won't sit well." I fabricate the truth. Yes, dyes bother me, but I don't know that I'm allergic to whatever is in that one. I just don't want to drink it.

"We could just do a food test," he says without questioning. "Eat a big breakfast then do a blood draw an hour after your first bite. It should tell us what we need to know."

I'm shocked at how easy it is to get him to waiver and cater to my needs. He truly is a blessing, and I'm so thankful that we found him.

Eggs, Toast, and a Doula

My diabetes test is tomorrow morning. I stand at the window of Blake's dance class, watching her pirouette across the floor, when a voice startles me.

"Did you decide on where you're having the baby?"

I turn to see Lena, coasting toward me with her youngest daughter on her hip.

"Hey! Yeah, I actually called the midwife."

"You did? That's great!" she exclaims.

"Yeah, but she can't do it because I'm high risk. So, she referred me to an OB who delivers out of the local hospital."

"Bummer. Do you like the OB?" she asks, pulling the stick out of her hair and allowing it to drop down.

I nod my head, "I really do. I was pleasantly surprised. I feel very calm with him. It's good so far."

She smiles back. "It's a shame you couldn't have a home birth. It really is incredible. But, it's most important to be safe and comfortable. I'm so glad you found someone that offers you that."

Talking to Lena is effortless. She seems to genuinely care about what I say and is quite educated about childbirth.

"How do you know so much?" I inquire.

She flips her hair back into a bun and shoves the stick through it. "Well," she starts, "I'm actually training to be a Doula."

"A Doula?" I repeat.

"Yes! It's like a birth coach. An advocate for the mother during delivery. Someone to speak for you to make sure your wishes are being followed when you may not be able to speak for yourself. It's really amazing. I love it."

A doula.

I don't know much about it, but it sounds wonderful. I could've used one in my first delivery—that's for sure.

"Do you get paid for this kind of thing? If you don't mind my asking."

"Yup. Once I'm certified, I can charge whatever I want. Most Doulas around here charge between 500 to 1000 for the whole process. From conception to delivery," she explains while she shifts her glance to her daughter dancing.

I'm eating up her words. Pure amazement fills my eyes.

"Can I get your number?" I ask as excitement overtakes my emotions. "I need to talk to my husband, but I feel like having a doula would be an amazing asset this time around."

"Absolutely!"

✳✳✳✳✳

The next morning I have my diabetes test. Shawn and I head to the local diner with Blake and a friend, and I order a two-egg omelet, two pieces of toast, a side of sausage, and a large cup of apple juice. Upon the first bite, I take note of the time. After ten minutes, the plate is empty and I hope it was enough food to show the results I need.

The nurse stares at me when I explain that I won't be consuming the vile juice she's trying to hand out. She reluctantly agrees to draw blood after reading the script from Dr. Paul.

"This isn't usually how it's done," she mutters under her breath.

I wrinkle my nose with displeasure. "I'm allergic to the drink."

She pushes down on my arm with a piece of gauze. "Your doctor should have the results in a few days, but I wouldn't count them as reliable. Let's just hope you don't have diabetes for the sake of your baby."

I exit the room before I say something I'll regret and head home to rest.

✳✳✳✳✳

"Your blood sugar was under 120, so that's good. I see you're set up for an ultrasound with Dr. Volgo next week," Dr. Paul reads off the paper in his hand. "Do you know what it's for?"

I nod. "They want to check the location of the placenta to make sure it's not covering the cervix anymore."

"Ahh, I see. Ok. Those things usually clear up on their own. A lot of placentas shift," he explains while he tightens the blood pressure cuff over my right bicep. "Almost 30 weeks now. How have you been feeling?"

"Oh, not too bad. Getting nervous about the Preeclampsia and delivery," I start. "Could we talk about it? Like a birth plan or something, in case I do go early."

"114 over 72," he says while undoing the cuff. "We can, but you're not going early. Your baby is going to stay in there until she's done cooking."

I smile at his ignorance. I like to be prepared, and I'm pretty sure she won't be in there the full 40 weeks.

"What would you like to discuss?" he asks as he takes a seat in front of me.

"I want a natural delivery with no meds," I explain.

He nods in agreeance. "It's your decision, and I support that. Are you ready for that?" he asks Shawn.

"She wears the pants," Shawn chuckles back. "I'm here to support her wishes."

"Smart man," Dr. Paul snips.

I roll my eyes, unamused. "Men," I mumble.

"I want a vaginal delivery. No episiotomy. Immediate skin to skin. Delayed cord cutting. Alone time with baby and family once we are out of any possible immediate danger," I continue to explain my wishes and Dr. Paul agrees to all of them.

"Do they have birthing balls? Or, birthing tubs? Or, maybe a squat bar?" I ask.

"I believe so," Dr. Paul responds. "We can deliver in different positions, but the hospital does not allow water birth. That's policy."

I'm disappointed, but I figured there would be some rules I would need to follow.

"I know you're afraid," he says while he places a hand on my knee. "You have every right to be. But, I'm going to take care of you. You will be fine. It's going to be perfect."

I smile and suck a deep breath into my lungs. The baby starts kicking as I lie back and await the sound of her beautiful heartbeat.

Swimming in Fluid

"The placenta looks great," the tech explains while she coasts the wand over my stomach.

"Your baby is measuring big, and your fluid is above the normal range. Did you do the diabetes test?"

I nod my head, "Yes, at around 26 weeks. My sugars were fine."

She prints out a paper and walks toward the door. "I want to show this to the doctor. I'll be right back."

I can feel the nerves build. It's like an elephant just sat down on my chest. Tiny needles prick me all over as sweat pours from my palms. "Babe, something's wrong."

Shawn lifts Blake off his lap and walks over toward me. "Everything will be fine, ok? Whatever it is, it'll be fine."

The tech returns with Dr. Volgo in tow.

"So, Ryan, your fluid levels are measuring high, and your baby is measuring above average for her age. Sometimes this can mean that your conception date is incorrect, but since she was measuring fine at the anatomy scan, we know that's not the case," Dr. Volgo explains.

My hands tremble. I grip the paper under them and crinkle it between my fingers. "So, what else could it be?"

"Well, we are thinking more along the lines of gestational diabetes. A lot of times it makes big babies and lots of fluid. I want you to retake the diabetes test."

The trembling stops. "Retake it? But, my numbers were beautiful? I have no other symptoms of it."

"Yes, that's true. But, there's really no other explanation, and it can have serious consequences if it's not managed correctly with diet or medication."

Medication?

I don't want to be drugged up. I also don't want to go through the diabetes test again. I absolutely refuse to drink that drink.

"No," I blurt out. "I'm not doing the test."

"May I ask why not?" Dr. Volgo asks. A very apparent condescending tone has now appeared in his voice.

"I won't drink it," I respond, firmly.

"You do understand that undiagnosed diabetes can cause complications?"

"Of course I do. I will watch my diet and monitor my blood sugar at home. I will bring you a print out of my levels at my next visit. It'll be more accurate than a one-time test anyway."

I'm impressed with my courage. Saying no to a doctor is not something I would've done six years ago.

"I suppose that will have to be sufficient. I will set you up a meeting with our nutritionist," he explains as he scribbles on the paper.

I wipe the gel from my stomach and shove the ultrasound pictures in my purse. I'm annoyed with the pressure for—in my opinion—unnecessary testing. Following Dr. Volgo out the door, he leads us to an office.

"Have a seat," he demands.

[130]

After twenty minutes of staring at my husband and listening to Blake whine in my ear about her boredom, an overweight, sandy-haired, middle-aged woman springs through the door.

"Well, hi there!" she exclaims, annoyingly loud. "I'm the nutritionist. Let's go over your diet options."

Let's not.

I roll my eyes, "I'm sorry, but I don't want to waste your time. I already eat very well, and until the diabetes is confirmed, I don't really think this is necessary."

"Nonsense," she waves her hand at me. "This will only take a minute. Here's a chart that lists good meal choices."

I sit back in my chair and zone out while she explains. My diet is clean. I limit sugars and grains already, and eat mainly protein, fruits and vegetables. I have zero interest in this information because I'm almost positive I do not have diabetes.

"Well, how about we go over the testing supplies. Most of it is covered by insurance. All you have to do is show them the bloodwork from your abnormal sugar level screening."

This is how they get you.

"I'm not doing the blood test," I inform her.

She looks baffled. "What do you mean? The doctor told me he's concerned you have diabetes and we are waiting on test results?"

"Perhaps," I begin, "but I'm not doing the blood test with that disgusting drink."

"I see," she says while closing her booklet. "Well, if you aren't doing the test, insurance won't pay for your supplies. You will have to pay for them out of pocket."

Of course I will.

"How expensive are the strips and things? My mother has a test kit I can borrow."

"Maybe around 20 dollars for a case of 100 strips," she responds. "Better if you don't need to pay out of pocket."

I nod my head, unwilling to waiver on the blood test. Receiving the packet of information she hands me, we head to the front desk to schedule a return appointment.

"Thank you for your time. I'll read over this stuff," I say as we walk away, attempting to exit.

The secretary at the front desk waves me down, handing me a slip of paper. "He wants to see you weekly for non-stress tests and fluid checks."

"Weekly?" I respond.

She nods her head without looking up. "Is next Friday at 3:00 ok?"

"It's fine," I say, exhausted.

We leave the office disappointed. I thought this pregnancy was going to be different; uneventful. But instead, here we are again. A different complication, yes, but still far from normal.

Did you say Free?

At dance the following week I inform Lena about my recent doctor visit.

"I'm so sorry this is happening. You know, some people just have big babies. Blake would've probably been between 8.5 and 9 pounds if you went full term. That's a good size," she explains while we sit next to each other in the waiting room.

"I brought you a book," she adds as she reaches into her bag. "It's written by Ina May. She's amazing. She is a midwife who lived on a farm where she delivered tons of babies, totally naturally. She's all about trusting your body and explains how to have the natural birth you want. I think it'll really help you."

I accept the book and begin perusing it as Lena continues talking.

"You know," she pauses to fix her hair. Sticking the bobby pin between her lips, she tosses her long-black pony into a messy bun—her signature move. Pulling the pin from her mouth and sticking it in, she begins again, "I was thinking about being your Doula. I mean, if you want?"

I close the book and stare into her brown eyes. We've grown close over these past few months, and I really do love everything she stands for, but it's just not feasible.

[133]

"I don't have that kinda money, Lena. I would love to have you there to help me through this. But, it's just not something I can afford."

"I understand," she responds. "That's why I'm offering it for free."

Her corner lip turns into a smirk. She pulls her legs up under her butt and turns to face me. Nibbling at her thumbnail, she awaits a response.

"You're serious?" I ask.

She giggles.

"I can't accept that. I love the offer, but I feel like it's undeserved. You don't owe me that. I haven't done anything to deserve it."

"Ryan!" she scolds. "You deserve to have the delivery you want. If I can help you do that, then that's enough payment for me. Let me do this for you. Please?"

I smile, "Ok. But, this means you'll have to see my lady bits and it will change our friendship forever."

She chuckles, "I promise to remain very professional, and can stand at your head for delivery if you wish."

The girls run out of class and we halt the conversation for now. Once home, I inform Shawn of the details. Hopefully, Lena holds true to her word, and I do get the delivery I'm wishing for.

✳✳✳✳✳

"Your levels are still high," Dr. Volgo explains at my 37 week scan. "I want to talk about a scheduled C-section."

"Are you kidding me?" I ask in disbelief. "Can you explain why? My sugar levels are fine."

"If she gets much bigger, you may not be able to deliver her. She could get stuck in the birth canal. High fluid can cause things like cord prolapse, or premature delivery. I want to deliver you at 39 weeks."

I'm fuming. I do not want a scheduled cesarean and I refuse to give in to his requests. However, fear begins to cloud my judgement.

"What's a cord prolapse?" I inquire.

"Well, if your water broke and the baby was floating above the cord, it could slip out before the baby. Then it would become compressed by the baby's head and the blood supply, and oxygen, and everything baby needs, would be cut off."

"So, the baby would die?" I ask.

"Probably," he responds. "Or, brain damage, at least."

I've learned how things work in life. People have their own agendas. They have sales pitches to suit them and to manipulate things into what they want. Sometimes, unfortunately, doctors are no exception. I need to explore if this is a real threat, or if it's just another agenda.

"I'm going to talk to Dr. Paul about all of this and get back to you," I explain.

Dr. Volgo is annoyed, yet again. He hates when I don't agree with his requests, but it's not his baby. It's mine.

"I think it's dangerous to go past 39 weeks. I'll send my requests along to Dr. Paul. I'm sure he will agree."

Even though I feel attacked, I choose to say nothing else as I head out the door. My appointment with Dr. Paul couldn't come soon enough.

You're Going Where?

"No, we're not doing a scheduled induction or cesarean. I see no reason," Dr. Paul explains to me as he looks over the paperwork from Dr. Volgo.

"Thank goodness," I reply. "I really want to let the baby come naturally."

"Yes," he responds. "Now, I will be away until the 9th."

I feel like someone kicks me in the back and can't catch my breath. "You're what?"

"I have a family trip I'm taking for two weeks. I have other doctors that cover for me while I'm away. If you go into labor before I return, one of them is going to deliver you."

"No," I blurt out. "I did this to have you. That was the whole point of a private doctor; a single practice. I don't want a stranger delivering my baby."

Dr. Paul sits on the chair and rolls over to me. Staring into my eyes through his black-rimmed glasses, he whispers, "Keep her in until your due date and you won't have to worry. I'm positive I will be here for your delivery. Now, are you?"

I rub my sweat-soaked hands on my shorts and try to formulate a sentence. I am convinced that this baby is coming early. If there was a way to bet on it, I would. I nod; knowing very well that he won't be there for me, and that—once again—a stranger will be delivering my daughter.

I sulk out of the appointment, and remain speechless the entire ride home. There really is nothing to say. It's been almost 38 weeks of pregnancy and my due date is closing in. Fear and uncertainty have begun to trickle back into my mind. The one thing I didn't worry about was having a doctor whom I trusted. Now, the rug has been pulled out from under me. There are no words to describe the pool of despair I am feeling—Dr. Paul has failed me.

"Let's reach out to those doctors covering for him," Shawn says from the driver's seat. "Maybe we could meet with them? Brief them on your history?"

I stare out the window. "No, I don't think so."

✳✳✳✳✳

"Lena, can you come over?" I ask through the telephone. "I can't tell if my water is leaking or I'm peeing myself.

I expect a giggle, but instead I'm met with a stern professional voice.

"Absolutely. I'll be there in 15 minutes. Stay calm."

Deep breaths follow as I study the wet spot in my underwear before putting on a new pair. Every time I stand, more seeps out, coating whatever fabric it contacts.

Shawn is at work. I'm only 38 weeks and have had no real contractions, only Braxton Hicks, up until this point. He will stay there unless I'm in labor. No sense using a vacation day if it ends up being a false alarm.

Lena arrives after several underwear changes. I sit on a towel in the living room, hoping she has some wisdom to offer.

"Hey Ryan, how are you feeling? Any noticeable contractions?"

I shake my head. "How do I know if it's my water? Will I get an infection? Should I call the doctor? My doctor is away for another ten days."

"Take a deep breath, Ryan," she starts as she sets her purse down on the table and meanders over toward me. "Let's figure this out together. First, if it was your water it would be a constant leak. Let's try to lie on our side and stand up."

I do as she says. Upon standing, I feel the familiar wetness in my underwear again.

"If it's not weird, smell it," Lena instructs. "Your amniotic fluid should smell sweet."

Pregnant women are a different breed. I run to the bathroom to smell my wet panties before Lena even finishes explaining.

No scent besides sweat. It's the end of June, and I'm a beached whale—sweat is an understatement. But, I'm still worried. It seems like an awful lot of wetness for just sweat.

"I think I'm gonna call the doctor. I'm just worried about infection," I explain to Lena.

She hands me the phone. "Maybe it's best if you get checked just to make sure."

I put a call into the office and the on-call OB returns it within minutes. I briefly explain my symptoms and history, and he directs me to head to the hospital to get checked. If it is my water, he will induce me.

I throw a few things into my already-packed hospital bag. Mom pulls in the driveway as Lena and I finish locking the door. I text Shawn while I buckle my seatbelt and worry about what's going to happen in the next few hours. The thought of coming home with a premature baby again is overwhelming. I fight panic attacks the entire journey— Deja-vu hits me as I remember the ride all those years ago on these same roads.

*****

Upon arrival, they direct me to triage. The resident OB has been briefed by the doctor I spoke with and is quick to prepare for a cervix check.

"So, you think you're leaking fluid? How far along are you?"

She lifts the paper covering my bottom half while three nursing students stand behind her, staring at my vagina. I try to answer her questions, but my brain is having trouble focusing.

Lena senses my hesitation. "She doesn't want students present during exams, please," she commands. "This is really something that should be asked, not implied."

I'm so thankful that she spoke up so I didn't have to. The students are baffled and unsure of whether they should stay or leave.

"Yes, of course," the resident complies as she waves them out the door. "Ok, so your amniotic sac seems intact. You are starting to dilate. You're about a centimeter, or so."

"What's that mean? Not much longer, right?" I ask anxiously.

"Doesn't really mean anything," she responds. "You could be three centimeters for weeks, or you could be nothing and have the baby today. It's really no indication."

Well, that's not helpful.

She finishes the exam and explains what to watch for and how to tell if I am, in fact, leaking fluid.

"I think it's probably just urine," she says.

How embarrassing. I've simply been peeing myself this entire time.

Lena stands at my shoulder. "It's good, Ryan. Keep that baby in there until she's ready. More chance of your doctor being back for the delivery."

I slide into my pants and prepare to leave when the nurse stops me.

"Have you done your pre-labor check in and tour yet?" she asks.

"No, not yet," I respond. "I actually have my appointment scheduled for later today to go over my birth plan and medical history. Stinks because I live over an hour away, I guess I'll have to find something to do for a while; pointless to drive all the way home."

[140]

"Let me call Julie and see if she can fit you in quick, then you don't have to come back later."

"That would be amazing," I say with excitement.

A few minutes later the nurse returns. "Great news, she can do a quick phone interview with you to discuss your birth plan and medical history. It'll take about five to ten minutes. Would you like to do that now before you leave?"

"Yes, please. That would be great!"

I grab the phone from the nurse and say, "Hello?"

"Hi, Ryan. This is Julie from the labor and delivery intake office. I want to ask you a few questions, if that is ok?"

"Yes, that's fine."

"First, is this your first baby?"

"No, this is my second. I actually delivered my first baby here with you guys about six years ago. You should have my paperwork on file."

"I looked, and couldn't find your name. Is there a different name you may have gone by? Perhaps, a maiden name? Did you get married since then?"

"Yes, I'm sorry. I didn't even think about that," I reply.

As she searches for my file, I answer a few more questions about my first pregnancy and medical history.

"Ok, Ryan, now let's talk about your birth plan. I'm not sure about your stance on all of these, but the hospital is strongly pushing for more parental involvement. We prefer that mothers try to keep their baby with them immediately after birth, and are involved in the infant's first bath and measurements. Also, we encourage all moms to breastfeed. We have lactation consultants on staff to help you with that if needed."

Are you serious?

"That is so good to hear," I respond. "I will definitely be breastfeeding. I'm glad you have decided to encourage that more in your hospital. I felt very disappointed with my first baby because of the lack of reassurance I received while here."

[141]

She spouts off apologies, "I'm so sorry that you felt that way with your first delivery. Yes, we are trying to make our labor and delivery more geared toward the mother and baby relationship. We want to form that bond between them, right off the bat. We are actually in the works to get rid of our nursery at some point. We think the baby should be with its mother from the beginning."

Although I agree with what she's saying, I'm not sure I would've been able to take care of Blake without the help of the nursery and the NICU. I was exhausted, and it wouldn't have been safe. I'm not sure completely eliminating the nursery is wise, but I keep my concerns to myself.

"Are there any other questions you have, Ryan?" she asks.

"I don't think so," I respond. "I'm sure I will think of something later, though."

"Well, the nurse will give you a paper with my number on it. If you think of something else, just call me. I hope you have a beautiful remainder of your pregnancy and a fast and healthy delivery. We are so glad you chose our hospital and hope that we meet all of your expectations. Take care."

"Thank you, bye."

The nurse hands me some paperwork I need to bring home and fill out before delivery. Lena grabs my purse from the chair and follows me out the door.

"Did you ask her about laboring in a tub, like you wanted?"

Crap.

"No, I knew I forgot something. I'll have to call her some other time."

I'm so thankful that things are already going to be better. Breastfeeding won't be an endless fight this time, and I get to keep my baby with me in the room. Maybe I will get the delivery I'm hoping for.

Three Days... Again

It is July 12th—my due date—and I have gone from wishing the baby would stay in, to begging her to come out.

[There's this magic to pregnancy. The ability to carry a child in your womb is something that not every woman gets the chance to do. It's incredible to be given that gift, and I'm so thankful that I got the opportunity to do it twice. However, when your due date comes, and you haven't shaved your legs or seen your feet in weeks, you're ready for it to be over.]

I am overly ready and secretly hoping that today is the day. Mild contractions have been coming and going since I woke up, but they aren't anything to get excited about. My stomach tightens and tiny knives stab into my abdomen causing me to halt—a few moments later it passes, and I go back to cleaning the kitchen. I convince myself that they are no more than Braxton hicks and that my baby is going to live in my uterus forever.

I bounce on my giant blue yoga ball in the living room. The television flickers in the background with some cooking show, but I choose to focus on Blake playing in the sprinkler outside. She runs through the mud and laughs hysterically as the tiny streams of icy water splash her in the stomach. I can't imagine loving another

[143]

human being as much as I love her. This baby will have to accept that fact.

How can you love two children equal amounts? All parents lie; they have to. They must have a favorite, and I know Blake will be mine.

A contraction jolts me out of my daydream, halting my bouncing. The pain is sharp and starts in the front, but quickly radiates to my spine. This one is intense, and I'm beginning to remember what labor pains really felt like all those years ago.

"Hey, chica, you ok?" Lena asks as she walks through the front door.

I ignore her until the pain begins to fade.

"Contraction?" she wonders.

I nod. "I've been having them all morning, but nothing like this one. This was intense."

She sets her bag down on the chair, and then places her hands on my stomach. "Have you been timing them?"

"No, not yet."

"Well, let's see when the next one comes. Until then, try to relax."

I bounce on the ball for hours. Lena times the contractions that are steadfast at 12-15 minutes. Some are strong, some aren't. But, they seem to be consistent.

"I think it's early labor," Lena explains as she runs her fingers through her long black hair staring at the ends, plucking the split ones away. "Unfortunately, this phase is usually the longest."

I push off the ball and head to the kitchen to thaw meat for dinner.

Blake yells from outside, "Mommy! Towel please? It's cold."

I waddle one out to her, and hold her for just a moment while I wrap it around her shivering body. My belly pushes into her as she turns to kiss it. She has so little time left as an only child, and as excited as she is, it's going to be quite a change.

[144]

Another contraction forces me to bend forward, clutch my abdomen, and focus on my breathing. Lena rushes over.

"Breathe through it," she instructs as she massages my lower back. "Should be easing up soon."

Mom pulls in the driveway with pizza just as my contraction is ending.

"Figured you didn't feel like cooking. Wanted to make sure you ate, just in case you deliver tonight."

It's a nice gesture, but contractions are making me grumpy.

"Just put it inside. Blake can eat. Shawn will be home soon."

Blake takes off like a bullet, sniffing the pizza box on the way inside.

"I'm hungry!" she tells grandma. "I was running in the sprinkler."

While Blake is entertained, I walk around the yard with Lena for a little while longer. The grass feels good between my toes, and the vitamin D from the sun helps boost my mood. If this is the beginning, it's going to be a long night.

The contractions become steadier and my bowels are loose. All signs pointing toward delivery. I figure I will be in that small percentage of women who actually have their babies on the due date.

Wishful thinking, I'm sure.

Hours later, it's nearing midnight, and we sit in the living room, awaiting the next contraction. In fear of my water breaking, I insisted that Shawn blow up the air mattress immediately upon arriving home. I never did purchase a waterproof protector for our bed, and I'm regretting it. I never thought I would make it to full term this time, so I never expected to need it.

Three more hours pass and the contractions hold steady at twelve minutes apart. I walk the hallway to help move things along. I'm so desperate to get this baby out of me, that for hours, I pace the wood floors, hoping they will intensify with every step—assuring myself that if I keep moving, this baby will simply fall out of my uterus.

At four o'clock— without any warning—they stop.

[145]

Lena is fast asleep on the couch, and Blake is snoring on the air mattress. Exhausted, and a bit relieved, I curl up next to her and drift to sleep, wondering what tomorrow will bring.

The sun rises the next morning and my uterus is surprisingly calm. Besides the baby kicks periodically, nothing else is occurring. There is no sign of labor; not a single contraction. I roll over and stare at Blake as she peacefully dreams. Her tiny eyes flutter and her lips break open to let out minuscule breaths of air. She is beautiful— my greatest accomplishment.

Tears fill my eyes as I think about it.

What if something happens to us during delivery and she has to live without me? This could be one of our last days together. Why did I do this to her? Why take this chance? What a stupid, selfish decision!

Shawn whispers through the silent house, "What's going on in that head of yours?"

"I'm afraid, babe. What if something happens to me, or the baby? I can't leave her without a mom."

He spreads open his arms and welcomes me onto the couch. I sneak off the mattress without waking Blake and break down in his arms.

"It will be ok," he starts. "This pregnancy has been so different. Everything has been amazing and I think the delivery will be just fine. I know it's hard not to worry and not to dwell on the past, but you have to think positive. It scares the hell out of me, too. But, I have faith that it will be ok."

I lean into his bare chest and allow tears to fall down my cheeks and slide onto his skin. He wipes my eyes with his thumb before kissing the top of my head and pulling me in. I'm almost relieved in the break from contractions. It gives me time to prepare myself mentally. I didn't realize how damaged I still am after all these years.

✳✳✳✳✳

My phone rings at five in the morning, two days after my due date.

"She's in labor—we are on our way to the hospital!" my brother exclaims.

"Oh my! That's amazing! Send me a picture. Good luck!" I scream back.

Upon hanging up, my phone immediately rings again. This time my mother is on the other end.

"How are you? Any contractions? When do you think the baby is coming? Can I make it to Virginia and be back for your delivery?"

So many questions that I have no answers for.

"I don't know," I respond. "If you want to go, then go."

My sister-in-law and I always knew this would be a possibility. Our due dates were only two days apart. We had it in our minds that maybe we would end up delivering on the same day, and my mother would be distraught over which baby she would see enter the world. However, I always knew I would deliver early and that this wouldn't be an issue. Yet, here we are, and now I'm not exactly sure what to say.

Emotions flood my body. I don't want her to go— I want her here. I want her to stay with me. But, I know she wants to be there for both of us. I feel guilty denying her that privilege and opportunity. Maybe she could make it there and back. Maybe somehow she could be at both.

"Let me call Rachel and see what she says. It'll take me four hours, at least, to get there. I might not even make it," she spits out and then hangs up the phone.

I stare at the ceiling. Jealousy overtakes my body. I am *her* daughter and this is where she belongs.

The phone rings again. I answer, ready to lay into her.

"I'm not going. She's already dilated to seven centimeters. It won't be much longer. I'll never make it. And, I don't want to chance missing your delivery too."

A sigh of relief escapes. My sister-in-law is blessed with quick labors. Her first was only seven hours and it was an induction. This one ended up rounding out at about five from the first contraction to the baby being born.

[147]

I'm envious as I drift back to sleep, hoping that I will get to meet our daughter soon.

Due Dates are Just Estimates

"She's beautiful," Rachel explains on the phone. "I'm sending you a picture right now. How are you feeling? Is today the day?"

"I don't think so," I respond, disappointed. "I think she wants to stay in there forever."

"Don't worry," Rachel says, sympathetically. "She will be here before you know it. Enjoy this time and rest, you'll need your energy."

"I will. Thanks. Love you guys. Give that baby kisses for me. I will keep you updated."

I'm so jealous that she is done with it all. She has her baby and I'm still sitting here playing catch-up. I never thought I would be the one left in the dust.

After breakfast, I start contracting again, but I'm not getting excited about it. They aren't painful, and I'm still going about my normal routine with very little difficulty.

"Maybe she isn't engaged in your pelvis," Lena yells to me from the living room. "Maybe try to do some stretches. If she's not engaged, you won't ever progress."

"What kind of stretches?" I ask.

"Well, you could try bouncing on your ball. Maybe some deep squats. Getting down on all fours and scrubbing the floor."

I stare at her, soaking in her advice. At this point, I would eat fire if it would help—maybe I could smoke the baby out.

While bouncing on my ball, I search the Internet for ways to get the baby to engage in my pelvis. A lot of the things that Lena explained are on the page.

I read one aloud, "This says I can lift my stomach up and back during a contraction. Something about the position of the baby being too far forward. It'll put her head down on my cervix and speed things along. It's worth a shot."

Mom joins us from the kitchen with a mug of hot coffee in her hand. Blake plays outside in the yard, catching butterflies with her pink net and carefully placing them in her bug catcher. With every one she retrieves, she runs inside to show us.

"Let's try it. Next contraction I'll stand behind you and lift your stomach, then we will walk," Mom demands. "We are getting that baby out of you."

I do as she says. During my next contraction, we lift my belly and lean backwards. Although slightly uncomfortable, nothing feels different. I slip my flip-flops over my feet and we head outside. The July heat hits me as the door closes on the air conditioned house. My skin burns from the sun's rays. Waddling up the street, I halt and lift my stomach with every contraction. After an hour, and potential heat stroke, we decide to retreat to the coolness of the house.

"I give up," I whine. "I'm so tired. I'll just have to be induced Monday like Dr. Paul said. He won't let me go past 41 weeks, anyway."

Lena rubs my shoulders. "Why don't you go lie down and rest. Being tired won't help anything."

I ignore her advice and begin to cook dinner, hoping that the activity will spur on some stronger contractions.

By the time I'm done cooking, I have zero appetite. My feet hurt, but don't appear swollen. I head to the bathroom to pee while everyone eats, and decide to check my blood pressure.

[150]

"114 over 73," I read to myself. I still can't believe I've made it through with no signs of Preeclampsia. Maybe Dr. Paul is right. Maybe it really isn't going to come back this time.

After supper, Lena and Mom head home to rest. I insisted that nothing was going to happen anytime soon and would call them if I needed anything. Besides, Shawn has the night off work, so I'm in good hands.

By eleven that night, my contractions are light and consistent at ten minutes apart. I stare at the ceiling while Shawn snores in bed next to me. Exhaustion takes over and my eyes close, knowing that this baby is not ready to come quite yet.

✳✳✳✳✳

At one o'clock, I'm jolted awake by an intense pain radiating through my abdomen. I roll on my side, and tense my body, curling into a fetal position the best I can. I've had pain like this before, and it's been gas. So, I close my eyes and attempt to return to my slumber. Just as I begin to drift off, the pain returns. I sit up, slip on my shoes, and tie a robe around my belly. Trying not to wake anyone, I mosey out to the kitchen and pour myself a glass of water.

Soon enough, another pain hits me. Memories jolt back, and I realize they are contractions. Not the little flighty ones I've been getting the last few days, but real—dilate your cervix— contractions.

I pull out my phone and begin timing them; ten minutes apart and about a minute long. By two-thirty, Shawn realizes I'm out of bed and joins me on the living room couch. Together, we await the pain, timing them on our phones. An hour passes, and they are increasing in severity and consistency. I decide to call Dr. Paul to see when he wants me to come to the hospital.

"Have they been eight minutes apart for at least an hour?" he asks.

"Almost two hours now," I respond.

"I usually don't have people come in until they are five minutes apart. But, since it takes you an hour to get here, you can come down sooner. I'll have the resident check you when you get there and let me know."

I thank him and hang up the phone.

Emotions flood my body as I head into Blake's room to wake her up. Tears flow down my cheeks when I see the excitement in her eyes.

"Are you gonna have the baby, Mommy?" she asks.

"I think so, sweetie."

We embrace in a hug, and then I help her get dressed. Shawn loads the suitcases in the car and feeds the dogs before we leave.

I call Lena, and she agrees to meet me there. Her sleepy voice immediately makes me feel guilty.

"Do you want me to call you later? Like, after they check me, instead?" I ask.

"No way, lady!" she exclaims. "I'll meet you there."

Day one ... Again

"You're about three centimeters," the resident explains as she checks my cervix. "We can't admit you until you're at four. You are welcome to walk the halls to try and get things moving along. I can check you again in an hour."

I begrudgingly slide my pants and shoes back on and exit the room, shooting dirty looks at anyone who passes. I could've sworn I was at least five centimeters and am disappointed to learn that, even with the painful contractions, I'm progressing slowly.

First, Lena walks with me. We talk about the contractions, and her impending divorce. Thirty minutes pass and Blake joins us. We change topics and talk about the baby and how exciting it will be to be a big sister.

My mood lightens each time we pass the newborns in the nursery. There are three babies in there this morning—two boys and a girl. I watch them sleep, finding it hard to imagine that soon I will have one of my own.

Every new contraction is more intense than the last, and it's getting harder to talk through them. Once the hour is up, I head back to triage to get checked, convinced I must be at a six or seven.

[153]

"You're at four," she says, pulling her fingers out of my vagina. "We can admit you. Let's get you changed into a gown. I'll hook you up to a monitor."

I don't want a full-time monitor.

I begin to open my mouth in protest.

"She wants intermittent monitoring," Lena speaks up. "And, no IV for fluids. She will take fluids orally."

"Yes," I spout, thankful that Lena is strong enough to be my voice. "I want free range of motion, as long as it's safe for me and my baby. It's in my plan. Also, no pain medication or Pitocin."

The nurse makes a face of doubt and I melt into a hole of insecurity.

Maybe, I can't do it. She must know my expectations are unrealistic.

Sensing my hesitation, Lena whispers in my ear, "You got this, mama. Don't worry about what she thinks; she probably doesn't even have kids."

I correct my posture, and stand tall. "Please respect my wishes."

✶✶✶✶✶

Five hours pass and it's almost noon. Shawn takes Blake to the cafeteria for some food once she begins to whine in boredom.

Lena sits with me, rubbing my back during the contractions, unsuccessfully easing the stabbing pain in my spine.

"Sounds like back labor," she whispers to my mom. "I wonder if the baby is face-up again?"

I worry that this baby will be just as hard to deliver as Blake, especially if she's sunny-side up. It was part of the reason the doctor used the vacuum the first time around, but I'm not sure I would agree to all of that again.

I begin picturing the possibility of a C-section in my head before I'm interrupted by another painful contraction. They are getting more intense, and becoming impossible to talk through. The

[154]

only things soothing are making a low moaning sound and waving my hips back and forth. I probably look like an idiot, but I don't care.

As they build, I try to sit on my knees with my arms hanging over the back of the bed. The pain in my spine is unbearable. Knives tear into my bones. The blades twist and tighten the surrounding skin until it feels like it will split open. Tiny needles stab my hips and around my stomach, piercing every centimeter of skin and engulfing it with pain.

"It hurts!" I cry. Mom and Lena take turns pushing on my tailbone, trying to relieve some of the pressure, but the pain is too intense. "Can't you do something?" I scream.

Blake sits in the corner eating her bag of chips, unsure of what to do.

"Blake, why don't we see if we can get Mommy some flavored ice to eat in between contractions? It'll help her feel better," Lena explains as she takes her hand, leading her toward the nurse's station.

Shawn is now at my side, holding my hand and preparing me for the next contraction.

"About three minutes apart," he states. "They look pretty strong."

I know he's trying to be helpful, but I'm miserable. "I think I know that!" I scold him, and then immediately feel guilty. "I'm sorry. I love you. It just hurts. A lot."

"I know, babe. It's ok," he smiles.

For the next ten minutes, I'm attached to the fetal monitor. I can hear its humming increase when a contraction builds. I try to enjoy the breaks in between, but I'm too anxious about the imminent pain, that I forget to relax.

"Here's another one," Shawn says.

"Already?" I ask. "I just finished one."

"Yes, they are coming very close together. But, it looks like you get about three close together, then a nice break of a few minutes. Just try and get through this one. I'm right here," he explains.

I can feel my stomach begin to tighten, and I dread what's coming. The contraction builds, and I shift onto all fours, praying the position will ease the pain. Shaw pushes on my tailbone, but I swat him away.

"Please. Don't. I'm sorry. Hurts," I mumble.

He rubs my hair instead and tries to console me. Thankfully, the contraction ends quicker than the last, and I get a few minutes of rest.

Blake stands by my bed with a cup of lemon ice and a spoon. Her big hazel eyes are filled with concern. "Do you want some of this, Mommy? I could get it ready for you?"

I nod my head as the numbers on the monitor begin to creep up, yet again. I turn on my side and hope that my pain doesn't scare Blake. Breathing through my nose, I count in my head—one, two, three, four... hoping to keep it under control.

"I need to get out of this bed," I yell. The nurse is at my side, her blonde hair is familiar.

"I'll unhook you, you can try the ball if you want," she explains as she waits for my contraction to pass.

It's the same nurse I had all those years ago. She didn't remember me, but I remember her. My blonde angel—*Amy*.

I close the gown over my naked butt as I take a seat on the ball. Between bounces, Blake feeds me tiny bites of ice. The cold lemon feels good on my dry tongue.

Another contraction hits, and it's strong and long. Bouncing on the ball intensifies the pain, so I stand and lean against the bed. Shawn stabilizes me from behind, and Blake stands in the corner with a spoon of ice ready for me.

I don't feel pressure yet, but I'm convinced that I've got to be almost ten centimeters. These are too painful to go on much longer. I have to be close to the end.

"Can you have the doctor check me?" I ask the nurse.

It was now around one-thirty in the afternoon and I have been in active labor for a full twelve hours.

"He's actually on his way in now," she responds.

[156]

Dr. Paul rounds the corner as I take another bite of ice. "Let's see where you're at," he exclaims. "You look like you're doing well. Keep at it."

I lie on the bed and spread my legs, something that you get surprisingly used to at this point in your pregnancy.

"You're at about a five. I'm going to break your water. It should speed things along."

Lena rushes to my side, "You have a choice here. Are you sure you want your water broken? It puts you on a time limit and may not hurry things along. It's your call."

Although I'm thankful for her information, I go against Lena and agree to it, nodding my head. A balloon pops inside me, and I feel the warm liquid soak the bed. The nurse lifts my bottom and pulls the dirty pads out from under me, replacing them with clean ones. I know it won't be much longer now.

At this point, I have spent my entire labor in triage— a tiny room with one chair and a shared bathroom. The same room I started my induction with Blake in all those years ago. Bittersweet emotions flood my mind as I stare at my little Blake—who is not so little anymore. Soon, she will be a big sister.

The nurse keeps promising me that a room will be available any moment, but I'm not buying it. Actually, I'm not sure I even care. The only thing I can focus on is the pain. I want it over; I want it done.

"I'm afraid," I cry. "I don't know if I can do this!"

Shawn, Mom, and Lena rush to my side. Spouting words of encouragement in my ear.

"You can do this."

"It won't be much longer."

"You're amazing."

The nurse walks through the doors at three-thirty, and we finally move to a delivery room across the hall. I guess I should be thankful that I don't have to deliver my baby in triage.

Push, Push, Push

Once in the delivery room, I lie down on the bed. I'm exhausted and have no energy left to put into this labor. Dr. Paul meanders through the door and I pray I'm at ten centimeters. I need to push. This needs to be over.

"You're at eight," he explains.

I give up.

"Eight?! That's it!? I can't do this anymore. I can't do this anymore!" I yell. I have failed. I have completely given up hope at succeeding in the birth I had imagined. I roll onto my side just as another contraction hits.

Tears fill my eyes and I plead with Mom.

"Please, get me an epidural. I cannot do this."

Lena squats beside me. "Why don't we try to walk before you make any decisions? It might get you to ten faster."

I roll to my side and push myself off the bed. Amniotic fluid drips down my legs as I scream in agony. Every step is absolute torture. With one arm over Mom's shoulder and the other over

Lena's, I walk to the door. Shawn's hands support my waist as my legs buckle underneath me from exhaustion. I drop to the ground when the next contraction hits, unable to move. The hallway spins as we enter it and I try to shuffle my feet in front of one another, but the pain is too much to bear.

"Please?" I beg. "Please get me the epidural. I just can't do it. I'm sorry." Guilt is all I feel. I let everyone down—I let myself down I know they will be disappointed in me that I'm a failure.

"I'll call the anesthesiologist right away!" Dr. Paul exclaims. "She owes me a favor. I'll get her down here as soon as possible."

I love the words coming from his mouth. As much as I hated him ten minutes ago when he told me I was only eight centimeters, he is quickly rectifying it.

"Are you sure this is what you want?" Mom asks, knowing my birth plan.

"Yes," I respond without hesitation. "I want the epidural. I need to rest. I have no more to give. There's no way I'll be able to push."

Within minutes, the anesthesiologist is at the door. To my surprise, it's the same one that did my second epidural with Blake. I am thankful that it is her and not the guy, and I'm hopeful this time it'll offer me lasting relief.

She's grumpy. She has the classic resting bitch face that I remember so well, and I am not in the mood. However, she has the drugs—and I need the drugs.

"Hi there. You did my epidural 6 years ago," I say in my sweetest voice, forcing myself to smile through the pain.

Her grimace turns to a tiny smirk. "Is that right?" she asks.

She demands the nurse to pump a bag of IV fluids through me before she can administer the epidural. I will now be bed bound, and I'm welcoming it with open arms. The coolness of the fluids rushes through my veins, and I pray for the sweet relief of the needle in my back.

Ten minutes later, the bag is empty and the epidural is ready. I sit up, and clutch a pillow to my chest like an old pro. The nurse places her hands on my shoulders and asks my family to leave the room. A contraction builds, and it takes all I have to remain still.

I feel amniotic fluid run down my legs and onto the floor and wonder how there is still so much in there. The nurse glances down at her shoes as the fluid pools around them, but says nothing.

"Ok, you should start to feel relief within ten minutes," the anesthesiologist explains. "No getting out of bed."

I thank her and lie back. My left leg begins to tingle, and then turns heavy. My right remains normal, and I already know that it's not going to work as well as it should. Hopefully it offers enough relief to get me through.

Shawn returns to his position at my side. A contraction builds on the monitor, but I slip into a light doze. He smiles at me while brushing the hair from my face. The relief of the drugs is well deserved, because I'm so tired.

Blake climbs into bed with me, and cuddles in the nook of my arm. I want to sleep, but I fight it to enjoy the last snuggles I will have with Blake before everything changes.

Without realizing I fell asleep, I am awoken by Dr.Paul performing a cervix check.

"You're at ten, Ryan. Are you ready to start pushing?"

I stare at Lena, "What time is it?"

"Maybe around four, I think?" she explains. "You only rested about 20-30 minutes. Are you feeling pressure?"

I rub my eyes, "I don't think so."

The nurse explains how she didn't put a catheter in, but it's falling on deaf ears. I'm so focused on pushing, that I don't really care what else she has to say.

"Hold your knees with your hands and pull them back during a contraction. Bear down like you're going to have a bowel movement," the nurse instructs.

Yeah, lady. I've given birth before. I think I know what I'm doing.

A contraction builds and I push, expecting a baby to shoot out of my vagina like a waterslide.

"Nope, that did nothing," Mom explains.

Maybe the nurse is right. Apparently, I don't know how to push.

Two minutes later, I try again. Absolutely nothing happens.

"I don't feel any pressure to push," I explain. "I just don't think it's time."

Lena instructs me to relax while I can. It's not quite time to push, but it will be soon enough. The phone rings as I try and shift my weight onto my left side.

"Yes. Ok. Yeah she's pushing but not progressing. Ok. I can do that." The nurse hangs up the phone.

"That was Dr. Paul," she starts. "He got called into an emergency cesarean. He wants you to stop pushing for now. It may be a while."

I close my eyes and drift off again, welcoming the chance to rest. I could sleep for hours if these people would leave me alone. After what seems like five minutes, an incredible amount of pressure overtakes my abdomen. As a contraction builds, I bear down to push.

"Is she pushing?" Shawn asks from across the room.

"I think so," Lena responds as she rushes to grab my leg and hold it up. "You're feeling the pressure now?" she asks.

I nod my head. "I need to get in a different position," I explain.

Before anyone answers, I shift onto all fours. The numbness in my leg has disappeared and once again I will be delivering without the aid of an epidural.

I rip cords off my arms and throw them. The nurse struggles to reattach them before alarms on the machines sound.

"I'm so sorry," I tell her. "I'm just so sorry. These are in my way. I have to push."

Her face fills with worry. "But, Dr. Paul isn't here yet," she whines.

"Well, you better call him," Mom demands. "Because this baby is coming. I'll catch it if I have to."

[162]

I push through the contractions and can feel her moving down the birth canal. Fire burns my vagina. Knives rip my back apart. Tearing flesh and ripping nerves are the only things I can feel with each push. I squat on the table, my arms on the back of the bed and my knees underneath me.

Dr. Paul walks through the door. He rushes to throw scrubs on over his clothes.

"I want you to slow your pushing," he yells. "I need a few minutes here."

I ignore him. You cannot tell a woman in labor to stop pushing. I'm getting this baby out, and he better be ready.

After an eternity, he's dressed and at my feet. "Can you shift on to your back?" he asks. "I can help you more that way."

I don't want to. This position feels good.

Reluctantly, I do as he says. Immediately, he begins massaging my perineum to ease the baby through the canal. I can feel the relief it offers.

"I can see her head when you push," Shawn exclaims through tears.

"She's coming!" Mom yells.

I feel like she should be here. Every contraction is too much.

I cry in fear, "Something's wrong! Why isn't she out yet? I can't do it. I can't do it. I'm sorry."

Dr. Paul continues to massage. "Ryan, you are doing it. Just keep going."

"You can do this," Mom and Shawn encourage in unison.

I fall back on the bed. Complete exhaustion wins the fight and I give up.

"Take me for a C-section," I cry. "I have nothing left. I just can't. Please. Just take me in. Cut me open. Get her out. Please."

Tears fall down Mom's cheeks and I know I've disappointed her. I'm weaker than I thought.

"Ryan," Dr. Paul demands. "Three more strong pushes and it'll all be over. Now, let's go."

[163]

Why is he so mad at me? Does he think I'm doing this on purpose? Does he think I'm trying to be weak just to spite him?

"A contraction is coming," Shawn explains while staring at the monitor.

I don't want to do it anymore. I don't understand why no one will take me for a C-section. They don't realize how difficult this is. They have no idea what this feels like. I just want it all to be over.

"The only way for it to be over," Lena whispers in my ear, apparently reading my mind, "is to push this baby out."

As much as I hate to admit it, Lena is right. The only way for this all to be over, is to get her out of me. One, two, three ... I count in my head before throwing myself forward and pushing with whatever I have left.

"Ok, she's coming down. She's face up. You're going to have to push even harder to get her nose past your pelvic bone. Push, Ryan!" Dr. Paul yells.

"Push, push, push!" everyone shouts.

Tears stream down my face and violent sobs escape my mouth. I groan as loud as I can, hoping my voice will carry the pain away.

I feel her move down. Her head is finally emerging from my vagina.

"Ok, wait to push now," Dr. Paul instructs.

No. There is no part of me that is waiting. I have been in labor for days, and my vagina is currently expanded farther than it should be. I know one more push will get my baby out, and I'm not waiting.

I suck a final deep breath into my lungs and put every ounce of energy I can find into my abdomen. I push, counting to ten in my head. At four, instant relief sets in.

"She's out!" Mom yells.

"She's beautiful!" Shawn exclaims.

"You did it," Lena wraps her arms around my neck. "I'm so proud of you."

[164]

"5:02 pm."

And, just like that, she's here.

As I stare at her lying on my chest, covered in vernix, blood, and amniotic fluid, Shawn lifts Blake on his hip to help cut the cord.

Tears have formed rivers down my fiery cheeks as every emotion floods my core. Nothing hurts anymore as euphoria sets in. Her tiny hands clasp the skin on my chest, and her little eyes gaze around the room. She is absolutely perfect.

"She pooped on you," the nurse exclaims. "Let me get that cleaned up."

I laugh as Dr. Paul works to deliver the placenta.

"You have quite a bit of bleeding," he explains. A sense of worry fills his voice, and I can see the concern in his face. "I can't tell where it's coming from. Turn on the Pitocin."

The nurse clicks a button behind me and— without my consent— Pitocin pumps through my veins, forcing my uterus to contract. I'm too busy soaking up my newborn to even care about the drug I was so strongly opposed to.

"It's a vein in your labia. I need to stitch it," he explains. "I don't have anything to numb you. I need to get the bleeding under control. You need to try and hold still."

"Nothing to numb her?" Shawn asks. "What about the epidural?"

"It's worn off, and pressing the button won't get it in her system fast enough. She has to do it without pain meds. It has to be now," Dr. Paul explains sternly.

I nod my head, hesitantly agreeing to his wishes. I'm fearful, but I trust his judgement. The moment the cold metal pierces my skin, I want to jump out of bed. I feel everything; from the second the sharp end cuts the skin. The cold metal slides through the inside of my skin as the thread follows behind. Nothing is left to the imagination. Every ounce of pain you can imagine with this procedure, I am feeling.

It hurts worse than any piercing or tattoo I've ever gotten. The nurse peels Fallon from my chest and puts her on the scale while I wince away from the pain. Clutching the bed rails in my hands, I apologize to Dr. Paul profusely. I know I'm not sitting still and that this is potentially a life threatening situation.

He doesn't acknowledge my apologies. His intense focus on the issues worries me.

"Am I going to be ok?" I ask.

He ignores me again. "I need more gauze," he yells to the nurse.

I stare at the table behind him where blood-soaked pads lie haphazardly. One falls to the floor as he tosses another on the pile. His gloves and arms are stained in red, and I begin to feel weak.

"I got it stopped," he explains with a sigh of relief. "That was scary for a moment. It was a big vein. Tore it right in half."

He applies an ice pack and covers me with a blanket before leaving to deliver the lady next door.

"Busy day," he winks. "I'll be back to check on you in a little while. You're in the clear. Don't worry. Just get some rest and enjoy that little beauty queen."

It all happened so quickly that I never got time to panic. My legs shake from pure exhaustion as I struggle to slide back on the bed into a sitting position. Shawn grabs me under the arms and places me where I want to be with very little trouble.

The nurse places Fallon on my chest, and I pull my shirt down exposing my left breast. It tingles as she latches on and begins to suckle like a professional.

"Nine pounds—ten ounces—and 22.5 inches long. You are a miraculous woman," the nurse congratulates me. After checking my vitals, she leaves the room, giving us some precious time alone with our newborn.

Blake stands next to me, her eyes wide. "I love her, Mommy," she whispers in her tired little voice. "That was scary," she says. "You were yelling. I hid under the blanket."

A giggle sneaks out of my mouth, and I wrap my free arm around her pulling her into my side. I was wrong. I didn't have to share my love between my two babies. Somehow, I have even more love to give. I know it's been an incredibly long journey getting here, but I wouldn't have done it any other way.

For the rest of the night, I cuddle with my two babies. As they drift off to sleep in my arms, I breathe in their hair, soaking up this moment. I am so incredibly thankful for my children, and I don't take one single second for granted.

Recovery

"I need to pee," I inform the nurse soon after she returns. "Like, now. Can you help me?"

She unhooks me from the IV fluids and assists me to my feet. They are shaky, and feel extremely unsteady. I reach for Shawn and he rushes to my side. Lena holds Fallon in her arms, singing to her as I slowly meander to the restroom.

Sitting on the toilet, I wait for it to come. The nurse stands beside me, staring.

"I have to do number two," I explain, embarrassed.

"I can step out if that makes you more comfortable?"

"Yes, please," I respond. "I'll pull the string if I get weak."

She nods and exits, leaving the door open a crack and standing just outside of it. Upon finishing, only a small amount of urine escaped my bladder, and I still feel a strong urge to go.

"Is it normal to feel like this?" I ask.

"I don't know," she says. "Probably?"

She doesn't know? What the hell does that mean?

I return to my bed, and she crosses things off her list. Another nurse pushes on my uterus to check if it has shrunk correctly and a pool of fluid gushes onto the bed.

"Is that normal?" I ask.

"Yes, it's just the leftover stuff from the pregnancy making its way out. It'll last a few weeks, but should lessen every day. Do you forget from your previous pregnancy?"

Do I forget? Excuse me?

Her comment feels condescending, but I try not to take offense. "It's been a while and I had complications during recovery, I'm not sure what's normal," I explain.

She smiles, "I'm going to check your stitches. We have to watch for infection down there."

Before I can prepare myself, she pulls down my stockings and examines the area.

"Can you explain where he sewed me?" I inquire. "Was it like an episiotomy?"

She shakes her head, "Not exactly. You tore your labia, and part of your perineum. He stitched both."

"Your labia is what bled so badly, I guess you had some pretty big veins down there and one split in half," another nurse chimes in.

"Oh," I respond as my vagina throbs.

The nurse readies another ice pack to apply to the area, as an intense urge to urinate resurfaces.

"I have to pee."

"Again?" the nurse asks.

"I think so," I respond, embarrassed.

She helps me up and over to the bathroom. My legs are still unsteady as I grip the bed, and then the wall for stability. She slides the hat in the toilet to catch my urine before I fall down onto the seat. For a solid minute, pee flows out of my bladder, and I finally feel relief from the pressure. Warm liquid touches my bottom and I stop for a moment.

"Um, the thing is full," I say, pointing to the hat.

"Oh my," the nurse says as she helps me stand and dumps the contents into the toilet.

[170]

The urine is red, and I'm a little concerned.

"Is *that* normal?" I ask, for the millionth time today.

"It's a lot of urine. Didn't you have a catheter in?"

I can't remember. Did I have a catheter in?

"No," Lena yells from outside the door. "The nurse didn't put one in during delivery."

"You had an epidural, though?" she questions.

I nod as she helps me back on the toilet to finish peeing.

She shakes her head, "Anyway, your urine looks red because it's mixing with the fluid and blood from your uterus and vagina. It's normal, but we will keep an eye on it for clots."

"Oh, I know all about those," I chuckle.

A few minutes later, my bladder is empty and I feel much better. Shawn helps me to the bed, and Fallon is waiting for my breast. I hold her to my chest, and she latches on beautifully. The familiar tingle encompasses my nipple and I know we are going to be successful this time.

"Do you think I could shower?" I ask the nurse while she checks my vitals.

"Absolutely. There is even a chair in there if your legs are too weak to stand. Maybe your husband could help you."

I can't wait to shower, and as soon as Fallon is done nursing, I hand her off to Lena and place my body under the warm water. The feeling is incredible; by far the best shower I've ever had in my life.

"Mommy, can I hold the baby?" Blake yells through the open door.

"Sure, sweetie. Can you wait until Mommy is done in the shower?"

"Ok, Mommy."

Her tiny voice sends shivers of glee through me. I am so excited to see how she will be with Fallon.

After my shower, I apply an ice pack to my bottom and cover up with blankets on my fresh bed. Shawn sets Blake up with surrounding pillows before handing Fallon to her. Her face illuminates with happiness as she stares at her sister—so in love.

"I love her, Mommy," she whispers across the room.

My heart melts. Any questions I had prior to delivery about whether having another child was the right choice, have disappeared. I know that Fallon has completed our family, and I thank God that I made it through this pregnancy with very little hiccups.

Home Sweet Home

By Friday, two days after delivering Fallon, we are discharged. She is doing beautifully and nursing almost constantly. Shawn carries the car seat as we walk the halls of the hospital, reminiscing about all those years ago that we did this same thing. I sit on a pillow in the front seat, and feel the familiar throb of my vagina against the pad. I secretly wish I had taken a few ice packs from the nurse before I left.

Once home, Blake runs inside and colors a 'welcome home' sign for Fallon.
Shawn carries her into the living room and we take a seat. He hands her to me, and she immediately roots for my breast. My milk leaks from my nipple as it anticipates her needs. Breastfeeding has been like second nature this time around. I cannot believe how easy it has been and how well we are doing. I wish I would've been able to do this for Blake, and I hope that my milk will be able to satisfy Fallon for longer than two months.

"I want to go check my bleeding," I explain as I hand her to Shawn after she's done nursing.

Once in the bathroom, I pull down my pants and am surprised by the normal amount of blood soaking my pad. Hopefully I won't throw clots this time, and I'll be able to swim before summer is over in six weeks.

[173]

*****

"Has your bleeding stopped?" Dr. Paul asks as he examines my vagina for my six week checkup.

"Not yet," I reply, disappointed.

"Some women bleed for a while," he encourages. "Everyone is different."

The metal contraption clicks as it opens inside me.

"Everything looks to be healing beautifully, even your labia doesn't look bad, considering."

My poor labia.

I haven't had the nerve to look at my vagina since delivery. Quite frankly, I was afraid of what I might see.

"I'm gonna do a pap, and then I'll see you in a year. No news is good news on the results."

After he's done, I sit up and dress myself. Blake and Fallon wait in the car with Shawn as I schedule my yearly visit for 2016. I can't believe how quickly it all went, and how lucky I am to have gotten through this pregnancy after Preeclampsia.

As I say goodbye to Dr. Paul, he leans in for a hug.

"You did a beautiful job, Ryan. See? I told you it was a first pregnancy phenomenon. I promised you we would get through this together, and I held true to that promise."

Tears form in my eyes, and I wrap my arms around him. "Thank you, for everything," I whisper. "It's been one hell of a ride."

Shawn wipes the tear from my cheek as I slide into the front seat.

"Everything ok, babe?" he asks.

I flip down my mirror and stare at my two daughters holding hands in the back seat. Fallon's tiny eyes flutter as she dreams, and Blake stares at her with amazement.

"Yes," I reply with a smile. "Everything is perfect."

[174]

The end